Walking Together, Working Together

Edited by LESLIE MAIN JOHNSON &
JANELLE MARIE BAKER

EARLE WAUGH, *Series Editor*
Patterns of Northern Traditional Healing, volume 4

Walking Together, Working Together

Engaging Wisdom for Indigenous Well-Being

P Polynya Press   *An imprint of University of Alberta Press*

Published by

University of Alberta Press
1-16 Rutherford Library South
11204 89 Avenue NW
Edmonton, Alberta, Canada   T6G 2J4
amiskwaciwâskahikan | Treaty 6 | Métis Territory
uap.ualberta.ca | uapress@ualberta.ca

Copyright © 2022 University of Alberta Press

LIBRARY AND ARCHIVES CANADA
CATALOGUING IN PUBLICATION
Title: Walking together, working together :
   engaging wisdom for Indigenous well-being /
   edited by Leslie Main Johnson and
   Janelle Marie Baker.
Names: Johnson, Leslie Main, 1950– editor. |
   Baker, Janelle Marie, editor.
Series: Patterns of Northern traditional
   healing series ; v. 4.
Description: Series statement: Patterns of Northern
   traditional healing series ; volume 4 | Some chapters
   previously presented at conference Wisdom
   Engaged: Traditional Knowledge for Northern
   Community Well-Being (University of Alberta,
   Edmonton, 2015). | Includes bibliographical
   references.
Identifiers: Canadiana (print) 20220425272 |
   Canadiana (ebook) 20220428344 |
   ISBN 9781772125375 (softcover) |
   ISBN 9781772126228 (EPUB) |
   ISBN 9781772126235 (PDF)
Subjects: LCSH: Traditional medicine—Canada. |
   LCSH: Indigenous peoples—Health and
   hygiene—Canada. | LCSH: Indigenous peoples—
   Medical care—Canada. | LCSH: Well-being. |
   CSH: First Nations—Medicine—Canada.
Classification: LCC E98.M4 W35 2022 | DDC
   362.1089/97071—dc23

ISSN 1927-9671

First edition, first printing, 2022.
First printed and bound in Canada by
Houghton Boston Printers, Saskatoon,
Saskatchewan.

This book has been published with the help of a grant
from the Canadian Federation for the Humanities
and Social Sciences, through the Awards to Scholarly
Publications Program, using funds provided by the
Social Sciences and Humanities Research Council
of Canada.

Every effort has been made to identify copyright
holders and obtain permission for the use of copyright
material. Please notify University of Alberta Press of
any additions or corrections that should be incorporated in future reprints or editions of this book.

University of Alberta Press gratefully acknowledges
the support received for its publishing program from
the Government of Canada, the Canada Council for
the Arts, and the Government of Alberta through
the Alberta Media Fund.

We dedicate this book to our Elders, teachers, and mentors, to Indigenous Peoples and their allies who are striving for a healthier and more just world.

Contents

Preface

JANELLE MARIE BAKER

As an environmental anthropologist and ethnobiologist, I often hear Elders speak about how the health of the land is reflected in the health of people. In the academic world, research on medicine, health, and well-being are often quite separate from research on the environment and earth sciences. The authors in this book remind us that, in reality, our health and well-being is inextricably linked to the health and well-being of all life on the planet. We have to care for our local ecosystems in order to care for ourselves, and, in fact, the act of caring for the land, of being on the land and living respectfully, in itself supports our well-being.

My role in co-editing this book is rather like a set of bookends, as I was involved at the beginning of the project and then again at the very end. Leslie Main Johnson has been a friend and mentor to me since 2003, when she co-supervised my Master of Arts in Anthropology and then supervised my work as a tutor at Athabasca University until I had the honour of taking on her position and her courses as faculty at Athabasca University when she retired in 2018. During my PhD research in 2015, Leslie co-organized the Wisdom Engaged conference that resulted in many of the book chapters in this volume and in the earlier volume, *Wisdom Engaged: Traditional Knowledge for Northern Community Well-Being* (2019). I attended the conference in amiskwaciwâskahikan (Edmonton), and roomed with Fort McKay Elder Celina Harpe-Cooper (see Chapters 5 and 13 in *Wisdom Engaged*).

Celina and I have bunked together at Moose Lake in what is now known as northern Alberta several times. We have often laid in our bunks by the wood stove in a small trap cabin, telling stories and watching the northern lights. We worked together for years on a berry-monitoring project in Fort McKay's traditional territory, which is now also the region that has been excavated and surrounded by the oil sands mines in northern Alberta. I did not think twice about bunking together at a hotel across from the University of Alberta Hospital, where the meetings were held. The remarkable thing, though, was that Celina's daughter, who had chronic health conditions, needed to see her specialist at the University Hospital, and she came and stayed with us over several days while accessing medical care and supporting her mother on this trip to the city. At the time, this felt like so many trips to the city for meetings with northern First Nations co-researchers and friends, but now, in retrospect, I realize that the layers of relationships and well-being that we were meeting about were being enacted all around us.

This volume provides the reader with many examples of how, when research and community-based projects are based in good relations, well-being and conciliation can occur. I joined Leslie Main Johnson as a co-editor in late 2021, which for me has been a joyful collaboration and an honour to tend to the many voices in this book. While so many of us ponder how to decolonize academic publishing (McAlvay et al. 2021), the authors here do it clearly and well. The authority of an Elder sits well beside that of Indigenous community workers, Indigenous scholars, and academic allies. Many authors write about how Indigenous medicine and science-based medicine do not have to exist in an oversimplified dichotomy but rather in relation to patient and healer, community and the land. The lesson I learn from this volume is that we really do need to walk together to support one another and well-being for the sake of the planet and us all.

REFERENCES

Johnson, L.M., ed. 2019. *Wisdom Engaged: Traditional Knowledge for Northern Community Well-Being.* Edmonton: Polynya Press.

McAlvay, A.C., C.G. Armstrong, J. Baker, L. Black Elk, S. Bosco, N. Hanazaki, L. Joseph, et al. 2021. "Ethnobiology Phase VI: Decolonizing Institutions, Projects, and Scholarship." *Journal of Ethnobiology* 41, no. 2 (July 5): 170–91. https://doi.org/10.2993/0278-0771-41.2.170.

Acknowledgements

As editors of this book, we wish to acknowledge first the Elders, Wisdom Keepers, and other authors for their contributions. We need to acknowledge SSHRC for the 2015 Connection Grant and CIHR Aboriginal Program for the dissemination grant that enabled us to hold the conference that initiated this book. The tireless work of Elaine Maloney, formerly of the Canadian Circumpolar Institute, and of Dr. Earle Waugh, former director of the Centre for Health and Culture at the University of Alberta Medical School, was invaluable. We further acknowledge all of those who volunteered at the conference and who contributed transcriptions of the oral presentations, a number of which form the bases of chapters of this book.

Leslie would also like to acknowledge her colleagues who were then at the Alaska Native Tribal Health Consortium (Dr. Gary Ferguson, Meda DeWitt, and Margaret Hoffman David) for their vision and their aid at the conference, and for inviting her to Alaska to attend the Alaskan Plants as Food and Medicine conference in 2016, which enabled her to make productive connections, especially with Dr. Allison Kelliher. Thanks to Erik Visser and Glenn Eilers for helping to video-record Elder Harry Watchmaker's words, and to Riva Benditt for helping to cement a relationship with Harry and encourage his participation in the project. Dr. Eugene N. Anderson, professor emeritus, anthropology, University of California Riverside, read the entire manuscript of this book and contributed many insightful comments and helpful editorial suggestions. Dr. Chelsey Geralda Armstrong, now assistant professor of Indigenous studies at Simon Fraser University, also helped with some of the framing presented in the introductory chapter. The anony-mous reviewers, acquisition editor, Mat Buntin, and the University of Alberta Press committee provided helpful comments and suggestions. Thanks also go to Dr. Janelle Baker, assistant professor, anthropology, Athabasca University, for being willing to join the editorial team late in the production of this book and share her understanding of complex issues of Indigenous health, well-being, and voice. Thank you to Renata Jass for her editorial insight, and the copy edit team at the University of Alberta Press for their work on the manuscript. Finally, Leslie would like to thank her family for putting up with her during the sometimes-fraught production of this book.

1   *Building Pathways to Well-Being and Healing*

An Introduction

LESLIE MAIN JOHNSON

Considering Indigenous well-being in North America, referred to by many Indigenous people as Turtle Island, is complex. There has been a fraught relationship between settler colonists and the Indigenous Nations of this continent with many twists and turns since the arrival of European voyagers to the Americas in the fifteenth and sixteenth centuries and the incursion of colonial powers into the homelands of Indigenous Nations. Exchange of medicinal plants and notions of healing are part of this history, followed by the expansion of settler state power and the progressive marginalization of Indigenous Peoples, the spread of epidemic diseases introduced by newcomers, and national policies such as residential schooling (in Alaska referred to as boarding schools and in Canada as residential schools) and forced hospitalization for tuberculosis patients.

This book seeks to explore ways in which communities, Elders, and non-Indigenous institutions can work together to improve Indigenous well-being. Indigenous well-being must be considered holistically and includes mental, emotional, spiritual, ecological, and physical health. This broad conception of well-being entails understanding the relevance of many aspects of personal and cultural life ways, including access to traditional foods, artistic and spiritual expression, healthy interpersonal and social relationships, sources of cultural pride and identity, and culturally appropriate education and health care. Our geographic area of focus lies in northwestern North America, especially Alberta, northern British Columbia, the western Canadian Arctic, and Alaska. This book grew out of a conference with that regional focus held at the University of Alberta in February 2015, extending themes previously explored in *Wisdom Engaged: Traditional Knowledge for Northern Community Well-Being* (Johnson 2019), with a particular focus on collaboration between Indigenous people and medical and health care communities.

As of this writing, Canada is striving to grapple with the legacy of its colonial policies toward Indigenous Peoples whose homelands are within its borders. Since the final reports of the Truth and Reconciliation Commission (TRC) were released in 2015, attempts to figure out how to create reconciliation have reverberated throughout Canadian society. The roots of many of the challenges to community well-being, and to Indigenous communities in the Canadian provinces and territories, lie in the collective trauma experienced by Canadian Indigenous Peoples since the signing of the Treaties and the move to consolidate the territory of the Canadian state in the nineteenth and twentieth centuries, opening the way for European settlement and, more recently, for resource development in northern regions (Adelson 2005; Bombay, Matheson, and Anisman 2014; Greenwood et al. 2015). It is not my intention to review this history in detail here, but this context underlies the contributions to this volume, which collectively help to show ways forward—the face of reconciliation in action.

In contrast to the excellent recent volume *Determinants of Indigenous Peoples' Health in Canada: Beyond the Social* (Greenwood et al. 2015), this book does not start from a "social determinants of health" paradigm and seek to move beyond it, but instead is based in a holistic view of well-being that is culturally rooted, foregrounding cultural knowledge and conceptions of wellness, illness, and agency. This view embraces both Indigenous and cosmopolitan medicine, seeking complementarities and mutual engagement to promote well-being, health, and healing "in the round." Contributors to this book are Indigenous people, descendants of settlers, anthropologists, ethnobiologists, and healers. Some contributors are physicians, Indigenous and non-Indigenous, who are seeking to bridge cultural and conceptual divides to work toward integrated and community-centred well-being.

As Naomi Adelson (2005) has pointed out, the burden of historic trauma and social inequity underlies the substantial burden of poor health in Indigenous communities in Canada and in Alaska today. She highlights the mission statement of the Assembly of First Nations as reflecting this relationship between health and equity:

> We as First Nations peoples accept our responsibility as keepers of Mother Earth to achieve the best quality of life and health for future generations based on our traditions, values, cultures and languages. We are responsible to protect, maintain, promote, support and advocate for our inherent treaty and constitutional rights, holistic health and the well being of our nations. This will be achieved through the development of health system models, research, policy analysis, and communication, and development of national strategies for health promotion, prevention, intervention, and aftercare. (quoted in Adelson 2005, S46)

Many of the authors in this volume are actively involved in this process; they are on the ground, in their communities or partner communities doing research, communicating the results, creating models, and influencing policies, all the while grounded in cultural Protocols showing respect to Elders and Mother Earth.

During the COVID-19 pandemic, challenges in finding common ground between biomedical and Traditional Healing understandings have been thrown into high relief. In early May 2020, two things that exemplify these challenges came to my attention. In one, a news item reported that the RCMP (Royal Canadian Mounted Police) in Saskatchewan interrupted a Sundance Ceremony that was explicitly intended to address and bring healing to those affected by the pandemic because it did not conform to the letter of the public health orders of the province of Saskatchewan (Shield and Martell 2020). The other was an internet petition calling on Prime Minister Justin Trudeau to address fundamental inequities in access to health care and the ability of communities to conform to the requirements of social distancing and directives regarding hand washing on overcrowded reserves and places without adequate potable water (Banerji et al. 2020). The first speaks to fundamental differences in understanding of causes of illness and approaches to healing, while the second derives from structural inequities and marginalization of Indigenous communities.

A holistic conception of health, to be meaningful, must encompass *well-being,* not mere absence of clinical disease, as affirmed in the first clause of the Constitution of the World Health Organization (WHO): "Health is a state of complete physical, mental and social well-being and not merely the absence of disease or infirmity" (WHO n.d.). Moreover, efforts to improve Indigenous community health must take into account many factors, including historical trauma (Bombay, Matheson, and Anisman 2009), poor access to all types of government and health care services, and poverty. Lack of access to both traditional economies and contemporary employment opportunities, as well as dispossession from land (see, for example, Richmond and Ross 2009; Big-Canoe and Richmond 2014), exacerbate poverty and unhealthy diet through limited access to traditional foods and the high cost of locally available alternatives (Lambden et al. 2006). In addition to these factors, I would emphasize that conceptions of health and well-being are culturally rooted, and that access to culturally appropriate services, in concert with access to biomedicine, is crucial for appropriate uptake and effective healing. A recent trend to emphasize cultural safety in medical and service delivery underscores this point (e.g., Yaphe, Richer, and Martin 2019; Stewart and Mashford-Pringle 2019).

Bombay, Matheson, and Anisman (2009, 2014) and Elias et al. (2012) describe how multigenerational trauma stemming from forced relocation and enrollment in residential schools in Canada pervasively impacts health. In order to move forward with reconciliation and healing, we need a better understanding of historical trauma and its long-term effects (see also Marsh et al. 2015a, 2015b). The United States also had residential schools, usually referred to as boarding schools, with similar policies, connections to Christian churches, and goals of overt and explicit assimilation of Indigenous populations. These factors obviously impacted the health and well-being of the Indigenous Peoples of Alaska.

There is evidence that the retention of language and traditional foods is protective against some of the mental, physical, and spiritual health problems that result from the collective impact of trauma experienced during the colonial expansion of state power and ongoing dispossession and displacement from land (Oster et al. 2014; Chandler and Lalonde 1998, 2003; Royal Commission on Aboriginal Peoples 1991; see also Chapter 11 in this book). A number of studies have found that the close association of language and culture has a jointly profound effect on Indigenous health. For example, King, Smith, and Gracey (2009) write: "Language is crucial to identity, health, and relations...It is especially important as a link to spirituality, an essential component of Indigenous health. Throughout the world, Indigenous languages are being lost, and with them, an essential part of Indigenous identity. Language revitalisation can be seen, therefore, as a health promotion strategy" (78). The First Nations Health Authority explicitly recognizes this as well:

First Nations languages are rooted in our knowledge and values and they hold relationships to Creation, the land, identity, roles, family and community. This is why Knowledge Keepers and Elders say that working to revitalize our languages is one of the most important and fruitful ways to promote healthy and self-determining Nations, communities and people (Brown et al. 2012). Connecting to culture and identity by way of learning our language is also one of the best ways to break out of the cycle of trauma.

Although the importance of language is well-known to First Nations, the linkages between First Nations language use and improved health and wellness are also showing up in academic literature. For example, studies from across the globe are finding that people who use or have knowledge of their language have lower rates of diabetes, drug and alcohol use, and many other improved health outcomes (Adams 2019, para. 2–3).

A similar sentiment has been expressed by the National Collaborating Centre for Aboriginal Health (2016): "For Aboriginal peoples in Canada, who bear a disproportionate burden of illness, revitalization of culture and language is essential for improving health outcomes" (1).

The manifest impacts on the health and well-being of Indigenous Peoples in Canada and Alaska include language loss, cultural fragmentation, suppression of Indigenous spirituality and practices, concerted attempts to forcibly assimilate children through residential schools and separation from family, separation from land-based economies and traditional foods, removal of individuals from home communities and involuntary confinement in "Indian hospitals" (see Geddes 2017), and economic and social marginalization. These factors have impacted people and communities differently in different environmental, geographic, cultural, historical, and political contexts, so the particular challenges faced by each community are unique. In a broad brush overview, the settlement of Indigenous Peoples on reserves and through treaties in Canada's western provinces—Saskatchewan, Alberta, and northeastern British Columbia—differs substantially from the experience of Indigenous Peoples in the western Northwest Territories, the Yukon, and the rest of British Columbia, areas which largely lacked Treaty settlements. These experiences are distinct again from the experiences of Indigenous Peoples in Alaska, who are now part of the United States and whose history has been affected by the Alaska Native Claims Settlement Act (ANCSA) of 1971.

The contributions to this book by Alaskan authors show an interesting contrast in contemporary settings and avenues of collaborative care and promotion of well-being because of the different administrative and governmental context in Alaska, which was sparked by the discovery of enormous oil reserves in Prudhoe Bay on the North Slope in the 1960s. The desire to develop this resource was the impetus for passing the ANCSA and for the establishment of Native Corporations. The history of collaborative care in Alaska is thus distinct from that in Canada, and the emergence in 1998 of the Alaska Native Tribal Health Consortium (ANTHC) provides a different context for collaboration between Western biomedicine and Indigenous healing paradigms,[1] including a greater focus on nutrition from traditional foods.

Well-Being and Healing in Canada

Kirmayer and Valaskakis (2009) examine healing traditions and mental health of Canadian Indigenous Peoples, while Reading and Wien (2009) describe in detail health inequities and the social determinants of Indigenous health in Canada; these works clearly underscore the magnitude of the problems that need to be addressed. Richmond and Ross (2009) also examine determinants of First Nation and Inuit health. Their approach involved interviewing Community Health Representatives from a range of First Nation and Inuit communities who identified six determinants of health: balance, life control, material resources, social resources, environmental connections, and cultural connections. A critical concept developed in their article is that of *environmental dispossession*, which the authors define as "a process with negative consequences for health, particularly in the social environment," arguing that health research "should focus on understanding linkages between environmental dispossession, cultural identity, and the social determinants of health" (403).

As a response to the insights gained in Richmond and Ross's 2009 study, Richmond and her student Katie Big-Canoe went on to explore Anishinaabe youth understandings of the relation of Traditional Knowledge, language, and the land to health. The youth in this 2014 study felt that disconnection from traditional lands and the reduction of land-based activities and sharing were significant factors driving ill health in their community. They suggested a range of possible approaches to counter these trends and to reverse their negative social and health effects, including going out on the land with older community members, which Big-Canoe and Richmond (2014) called *environmental repossession*. They write:

> Based on the growing body of Indigenous scholarship oriented toward environmental reconciliation, resurgence of Indigenous Knowledge and way of life, and perhaps most importantly, Indigenous involvement in research, we offer the concept of environmental repossession as a way to frame these results. Environmental repossession refers to the social, cultural and political processes by which Indigenous peoples and communities are reclaiming their traditional

lands and ways of life. This concept is rooted centrally in the idea that
Indigenous peoples' health, ways of living, and Indigenous knowledge systems
are dependent on access to their traditional lands and territories. (133)

Terry Teegee (2015) also elaborated on the fundamental importance of the
connection between health and land, writing, "If you're really worrying about
and questioning your identity and your loss of identity, you're not a whole
person, and that really affects your health" (123). He further comments, "So
in many respects, the issue of land and our access to it, and our access to our
culture and heritage and language deeply affected how we are today and
where we're at today" (123).

A recent collaborative effort to enable urban Indigenous people to access
Blackfoot traditions and knowledge is chronicled in Victor et al.'s (2019)
"I'taamohkanoohsin (Everyone Comes Together): (Re)connecting Indigenous
People Experiencing Homelessness and Addiction to Their Blackfoot Ways
of Knowing," which specifically details the condition of Indigenous and
spiritual homelessness. The authors write, "Spiritual homelessness is a form
of Indigenous homelessness resulting from displacement from traditional
lands and kinship networks" (45).

The relationship of culture and health is taken up in an unexpected context
in "Technology, Material Culture and the Well-Being of Aboriginal Peoples
of Canada," (Guindon with the Neeposh family 2015), where they articulate
how traditional technology supports identity and well-being through cultural
competence on the land. After an articulate discussion of Cree terms for well-
being and an emphasis on traditional skills as a key way to live well, their
collaborative paper states, "The Mistissini are now determined to tackle this
'social suffering' [the legacy of residential schools and attendant poor community health]...with their own means. Various local institutions recently developed programs aiming to heal their community as a whole. Many elements
of their cultural heritage, including their technology, now participate in these
efforts" (88).

A similar holistic emphasis is clearly apparent in the descriptions given by
Mary Maje and Ann Maje Raider (Chapter 5 in this book) of the efforts of the

Liard Aboriginal Women's Society summer camps held at Frances Lake (Tu Cho Mene), Yukon, and its local programs in Watson Lake, Yukon, where hide processing, beadwork, preparing moose meat, camping, and spending time on the land are all activities believed to contribute to healing and the promotion of well-being. Likewise, Kaska scholar Linda McDonald (2019) argues strongly for the importance of language revitalization efforts and their positive effects on self-esteem and social well-being for Kaska.

There is evidence, as well, of a strong desire in Indigenous communities to move forward, to achieve appropriate access to health care that is rooted in both biomedicine and in Indigenous traditions. For instance, in a recent issue of *birth issues*, Nadia Houle (2017) makes a compelling case for improving Indigenous maternity care by reclaiming and improving access to traditional birth practices. She cites the Truth and Reconciliation Commission recommendations, and articulates the strong position held by Indigenous Birth of Alberta. In 2016, the National Aboriginal Council of Midwives also released a key report, *The Landscape of Aboriginal Midwifery Care for Aboriginal Communities in Canada*, which asserts that Aboriginal[2] midwifery care is widely recognized as "a best practice for maternal health care in Aboriginal communities across Canada" (3). The report continues by describing the decline of midwifery in Indigenous communities and states, "This has had a negative impact both on the preservation of culture and on maternal newborn health outcomes in Aboriginal communities across Canada" (3). The council contextualizes this by commenting, "It is widely acknowledged that infant deaths in Aboriginal communities are at least twice the national average" (3). Later, in the same report it describes Aboriginal midwifery: "Aboriginal midwifery is not limited to birth attendance and care during and after pregnancy, rather, the good health and well-being of Aboriginal women and their babies is crucial to the empowerment of Aboriginal families and communities" (5). The approach to reclaiming Indigenous power to pursue culturally appropriate care in birthing can be seen as resurgence. The ways we come into the world, and the experiences of families, new mothers, and babies in this process are areas where deep collaboration between the social, the cultural, and the medical can support reconciliation and healing.

In October 2017, Grand Chief Wilton Littlechild, TRC commissioner, lawyer, and former Member of Parliament, addressed the Integrative Health Institute Conference at the University of Alberta. To achieve reconciliation, he reminded us, we must ask: How do we restore respectful relationships? How do we heal? He asserted that the United Nations Declaration on the Rights of Indigenous Peoples, to which Canada is a signatory, must be used as a framework for reconciliation.[3] As a signatory, this means that Canada recognizes that international human rights law applies to Indigenous Peoples. Chief Littlechild stated that this includes a right to health. He also called our attention to the fact that numbers 18, 19, 20, and 21 of the TRC's (2015b) calls to action (see below) deal directly with Indigenous health. These calls to action, Chief Littlechild reminds us, are not speaking to needs but to rights.

Health

18. We call upon the federal, provincial, territorial, and Aboriginal governments to acknowledge that the current state of Aboriginal health in Canada is a direct result of previous Canadian government policies, including residential schools, and to recognize and implement the health-care rights of Aboriginal people as identified in international law, constitutional law, and under the Treaties.

19. We call upon the federal government, in consultation with Aboriginal peoples, to establish measurable goals to identify and close the gaps in health outcomes between Aboriginal and non-Aboriginal communities, and to publish annual progress reports and assess long-term trends. Such efforts would focus on indicators such as: infant mortality, maternal health, suicide, mental health, addictions, life expectancy, birth rates, infant and child health issues, chronic diseases, illness and injury incidence, and the availability of appropriate health services.

20. In order to address the jurisdictional disputes concerning Aboriginal people who do not reside on reserves, we call upon the federal government to recognize, respect, and address the distinct health needs of the Métis, Inuit, and off-reserve Aboriginal peoples.

21. We call upon the federal government to provide sustainable funding for existing and new Aboriginal healing centres to address the physical, mental, emotional, and spiritual harms caused by residential schools, and to ensure that the funding of healing centres in Nunavut and the Northwest Territories is a priority.

22. We call upon those who can effect change within the Canadian health-care system to recognize the value of Aboriginal healing practices and use them in the treatment of Aboriginal patients in collaboration with Aboriginal healers and Elders where requested by Aboriginal patients.

23. We call upon all levels of government to:
    i.   Increase the number of Aboriginal professionals working in the health-care field.
    ii. Ensure the retention of Aboriginal health-care providers in Aboriginal communities.
    iii. Provide cultural competency training for all health-care professionals.

24. We call upon medical and nursing schools in Canada to require all students to take a course dealing with Aboriginal health issues, including the history and legacy of residential schools, the *United Nations Declaration on the Rights of Indigenous Peoples,* Treaties and Aboriginal rights, and Indigenous teachings and practices. This will require skills-based training in intercultural competency, conflict resolution, human rights, and anti-racism. (TRC 2015b, 2–3)

Call to Action 21 speaks to the need to provide sustainable funding for Aboriginal healing centres "to address physical, mental, emotional, and spiritual harms caused by residential schools." Healing must include not just mind, body, and emotions. Spiritual health from a holistic perspective is important. Traditional medicine is also a very important part of the right to health.

In Alberta, reconciliation requires implementation of Treaty Rights to health. Treaty No. 6 has a "medicine chest clause" (1876), which has been interpreted to mean that Canada has an ongoing obligation to provide access to health services. This must go beyond the simple provision of medicines and medical supplies to ensure a state of health. Health is more than the simple absence of disease. It implies the right to well-being, as the WHO constitution emphasizes. The fiduciary duty of the federal government of Canada to Indigenous Peoples includes the responsibility to provide access to health care, but the inadequate health care provided through the federal system to First Nations, Métis, and Inuit communities demonstrates a long-standing failure of the Canadian government to meet its obligations: The sordid history of the Indian hospitals (Geddes 2017), as well as the inadequacy of the Non-Insured Health Benefits program (Reading and Wein 2009) attest to this failure. These issues have had widespread impact in the northern territories, as well as in the northern parts of the western provinces of Canada. We look to the TRC recommendations for guidance away from colonial violence and toward equitable access to culturally safe health care.

Building Pathways to Reconciliation

In the University of Alberta's 2016 Strategic Plan, it identified a Signature Areas Initiative[4] for which the university community developed a portfolio of research and teaching areas for global leadership. In a proposal to be included in the signature areas, the Integrative Health Institute (2017) wrote the following:

Relevance to Canada's Indigenous Peoples

Indigenous peoples (i.e., First Nations, Metis, Inuit) are among the most marginalized and underserved populations in the area of healthcare delivery. A key contributor to this problem is the lack of integration of Indigenous traditional health practices with conventional health practices. The resulting disconnect is recognized by the Truth and Reconciliation Commission of Canada and the World Health Organization's Declaration on the Human Rights of Indigenous people, prompting a call to "...those who can affect change within the Canadian health-care system to recognize the value of Aboriginal healing practices and use them in the treatment of Aboriginal patients in collaboration with Aboriginal healers and Elders where requested by Aboriginal patients" (TRC 2015b). Further, in May 2016, in accordance with the Canadian Constitution, Canada officially adopted and promised to implement the United Nations Declaration on the Rights of Indigenous Peoples, which acknowledges the right of Indigenous peoples to traditional approaches to health." (2)

Seeking collaborative solutions to these long-standing health inequities is an enormous challenge. Achieving health and well-being for Indigenous Peoples of Canada requires overcoming a huge amount of historical trauma (Bombay, Matheson, and Anisman 2009, 2014; Elias et al. 2012; Marsh et al. 2015a, 2015b) and dismantling the political processes of the colonial apparatus that have formed the nation of Canada (Napoleon 2013; Belanger and Lackenbauer 2014). On the process of reconciliation and seeking collaborative solutions, the commissioners of the Truth and Reconciliation Commission have written:

> Getting to the truth was hard, but getting to reconciliation will be harder. It requires that the paternalistic and racist foundations of the residential school system be rejected as the basis for an ongoing relationship. Reconciliation requires that a new vision, based on a commitment to mutual respect, be developed. It also requires an understanding that the most harmful impacts of residential schools have been the loss of pride and self-respect of Aboriginal people, and the lack of respect that non-Aboriginal people have been raised to have for their Aboriginal neighbours. Reconciliation is not an Aboriginal problem; it is a Canadian one. (TRC 2015a, vi)

Elsewhere, they continue:

> Aboriginal peoples have always remembered the original relationship they had with early Canadians. That relationship of mutual support, respect, and assistance was confirmed by the Royal Proclamation of 1763 and the Treaties with the Crown that were negotiated in good faith by their leaders. That memory, confirmed by historical analysis and passed down through Indigenous oral

histories, has sustained Aboriginal peoples in their long political struggle to live with dignity as self-determining peoples with their own cultures, laws, and connections to the land.

The destructive impacts of residential schools, the *Indian Act*, and the Crown's failure to keep its Treaty promises have damaged the relationship between Aboriginal and non-Aboriginal peoples. The most significant damage is to the trust that has been broken between the Crown and Aboriginal peoples. That broken trust must be repaired. The vision that led to that breach in trust must be replaced with a new vision for Canada; one that fully embraces Aboriginal peoples' right to self-determination within, and in partnership with, a viable Canadian sovereignty. If Canadians fail to find that vision, then Canada will not resolve long-standing conflicts between the Crown and Aboriginal peoples over Treaty and Aboriginal rights, lands, and resources, or the education, health, and well-being of Aboriginal peoples. Reconciliation will not be achieved, and neither will the hope for reconciliation be sustainable over time. (TRC 2015a, 184)

Legal and Treaty scholars Asch, Borrows, and Tully (2018) present a careful examination of the concepts of reconciliation and of resurgence, and of their interaction in *Resurgence and Reconciliation*. *Resurgence* is seen as a more assertive and equal approach to moving forward; "resurgence" foregrounds the value of Indigenous conceptions of the world and of relationships as necessary for both rapprochement between diverse groups of people, and of humans with other than human entities in creation of a socially and ecologically sustainable future.

The authors of this book hope to make a contribution to the resolution of some of the challenges to the well-being of Indigenous Peoples. In it, we examine a series of issues and cases that approach integration or collaboration of Indigenous traditional approaches to well-being, wellness, and healing with biomedicine and other approaches to wellness promotion and the treatment of illness. This is the face of reconciliation: working together across boundaries to heal communities, to promote Indigenous well-being, to explore ways forward. Topics in this book include Traditional Healers and their approaches to the treatment of disease and illness; integration of Traditional Healers and traditional medicines into the medical system; Traditional Knowledge and intellectual property issues around medicinal plant knowledge; querying the role of doctors as healers; Indigenous approaches to holistic wellness promotion in the Yukon, British Columbia, and Alaska; the role of diet and traditional foods in health promotion among Indigenous Peoples in Alaska; the potential of revival of women's rites of passage; innovative tools for women's healing in the Arctic through Photovoice; digital storytelling for healing; culture and diabetes incidence and effective treatment; mapping an approach to healing work with urban Indigenous populations in a respectful, collaborative, and culturally sensitive way; and integrating biomedicine, alternative therapies, and Indigenous healing in clinical practice. This book extends the discussion begun in *Wisdom Engaged: Traditional Knowledge for Northern Community Well-Being* (Johnson 2019), from the role and potential that Traditional Healing knowledge has in guiding community well-being in the North to examining how collaborative efforts to improve Indigenous well-being can be effective in the North and in the provinces.

Although the experiences of Indigenous Peoples in Alaska differ in some important ways from the experiences of First Nations, Métis, and Inuit people in Canada, the impacts of colonization have been very similar in both places, and the efforts made to take ownership of Alaska Native health services, prevention, and health promotion can help illuminate possibilities in Canada as well. Similarly, northern Canadian experiences may also suggest possibilities and ways to address challenges encountered in Alaska.

There are significant challenges to working across cultures and medical systems to enable integrative promotion of health, of well-being. Successful models are critical to move this endeavour forward. Creating spaces for open conversations about how to enable healing and promote well-being require a willingness to engage with distinct understandings of illness and wellness, and with health as a process, not a product. It requires looking for the ways that different understandings, standpoints, and perspectives illuminate the same phenomena, and seeing how understanding in the aggregate provides deeper knowledge than the view from any single perspective. It requires addressing well-being on a number of levels, encompassing physical, mental, spiritual, and emotional health, as well as individual, family, community, and environmental wellness.

About This Book

Several key terms that are fundamental to this book need to be addressed: Indigenous, Aboriginal, and Native. As of this writing, *Indigenous* is the generally preferred term to describe descendants of original populations in North America and throughout the world. Prior to the last few years, *Aboriginal* was widely used in Canada to indicate peoples descended from the original inhabitants of Canada. Prior to that, terms such as *Native People* were used. In Canada, "Native" was seen as having negative connotations and so was abandoned. In contrast, in Alaska, *Alaska Native* has been the generally accepted term, and is used in Indigenous communities, although *Indigenous* is preferred for description by outsiders. We have used the term *Indigenous* as the preferred term for Canadian Indigenous Peoples, and as a descriptor for Alaskan Indigenous Peoples. Where describing the contents of older documents and organizations in Canada, "Aboriginal" is used if that was the original terminology, while "Alaska Native" or "Tribal" might be used in describing institutions or organizations in Alaska where that is the original term used.

A note on methodology is in order here. Chapters in this book either originated as invited presentations for the Wisdom Engaged: Traditional Knowledge for Northern Community Well-Being conference held in Edmonton in February 2015, were solicited by me after the event to ensure representation of themes that were included in the conference but where presenters declined to submit papers for publication (Watchmaker; Kelliher), or were volunteered by a conference participant but not originally presented at the conference (DeWitt; Oster et al.). The texts of the chapters were arrived at through a combination of written submissions (sometimes accompanied by illustrations) and edited transcripts of oral presentations (some of which were accompanied by illustrations and/or photographs). All works were submitted by the authors as written documents, or, after reviewing and editing where desired, their transcribed words. Photographs were also reviewed by the authors or submitted by the authors, along with their written texts. Subjects of photographs signed consent forms indicating their agreement for their images to appear in the book. Authors reviewed their chapters again prior to submission of the final manuscript for copy editing, ensuring that contributors had full control over what is included in the book.

A note on language choices is appropriate here. We have chosen to retain Indigenous voice as much as possible in a written format. This means that the chapters contributed orally may have nonstandard written English phrasing. In addition, some words such as "Grandmother," "Grandfather," and "Elder" are capitalized to indicate respect in these texts. We have striven to retain patterns of Indigenous narrative form in chapters authored by Indigenous contributors, including chapters contributed in written form. In this we are guided by models such as that used by Métis author Maria Campbell.[5] We also include Indigenous words used in the texts.

The book begins with three short contributions by Indigenous authors from Alberta to introduce healing approaches that directly address collaboration of Indigenous ceremonialists and the cosmopolitan medical system. In Chapter 2, Cree ceremonialist Harry Watchmaker (Kehewin Cree Nation) expresses a holistic and spiritually grounded world view that foregrounds language, traditional foods, medicines, and Ceremony. We video-recorded his speech for transcription in this book and presented him with a copy to use in his ongoing healing work. Kainai (Blood) Sundancer and healer Camille (Pablo) Russell and his Tsuut'ina colleague Hal Eagletail worked in healing in collaboration with Alberta Health Services and Correctional Services. In Chapter 3, they discuss their holistic work to address the needs of their clients, tensions between knowledge systems and intellectual property issues for traditional medicines, and the history of collaboration of Indigenous healers with Alberta Health Services. Their presentation also embodies the healing role of humour. Finally, in Chapter 4, Darlene P. Auger, Cree from Wabasca, probes questions of the role of Western medical doctors in the healing process for Indigenous people.

Chapters by Mary Maje and Ann Maje Raider (Chapter 5) and Ruby E. Morgan (Chapter 6) describe two northern community-based efforts to promote holistic health and community well-being. Chapter 5 describes the efforts of the Liard Aboriginal Women's Society to promote healing and well-being among Kaska in northern British Columbia and the Yukon. Its efforts were funded by the Aboriginal Healing Foundation until that program was terminated. Then Ruby E. Morgan (Luu Giss Yee) describes efforts to implement a holistic community health plan based on Gitxsan principles in the western Gitxsan villages in British Columbia explicitly based on a collaborative approach that encompasses traditional Gitxsan wellness and healing approaches, alternative healing, and biomedicine. Both of these on-the-ground programs embody local community wisdom and vision, and they share a focus on the significance of culture and on-the-land activities.

In Chapter 7, Gary Ferguson, Meda DeWitt, and Margaret David present a review of activities and programs of the prevention division of the Alaska Native Tribal Health Consortium. This is followed by another contribution by Meda DeWitt, a young Tlingit Traditional Healer, reporting on an innovative women's healing initiative through establishing a Women's Rites of Passage encampment (Chapter 8), another affirmation of the value of on-the-land holistic healing. Chapter 9 shifts the focus northward, where Dorothy Badry (professor of social work) and Annie Goose (community Elder) present a Photovoice approach to women's healing and FASD (fetal alcohol spectrum disorders) prevention in Ulukhaktok, Nunavut. Chapter 10 (Marc Fonda) examines issues of intellectual property and Traditional Knowledge, and Chapter 11 (Richard T. Oster, Angela Grier, Rick Lightning, Maria J. Mayan, and Ellen L. Toth) articulates a collaborative effort between physicians and Indigenous collaborators to examine causes of diabetes in Indigenous communities in Alberta, looking for productive and culturally based approaches to reducing this health challenge.

In Chapter 12, family care physician Ginetta Salvalaggio examines ways of collaborating productively between health care providers and inner-city Indigenous communities, and she presents a useful model based on her pragmatic work in working with and treating inner-city residents in Edmonton. Finally, Allison Kelliher, Koyukon physician and Traditional Healer from Alaska, presents her story as a physician and healer and offers pragmatic approaches to healing based in the elements, plants, and traditional foods, drawing from Western medicine, traditional practices, and alternative therapies in an integrative framework in Chapter 13. I offer some concluding reflections in Chapter 14.

Seriously addressing Indigenous health disparities in Canada and the North is of necessity a process of decolonization, and it is in fact the face of and process of reconciliation. We hope this book is a small step along this path.

NOTES

1. For more on the history and mandate of ANTHC, see https://anthc.org/who-we-are/history/.
2. "Aboriginal" is the term used throughout this report.
3. The United Nations Declaration on the Rights of Indigenous Peoples speaks to fundamental rights that affect Indigenous health in Canada, and the relationship of Canada's Indigenous Peoples to other Canadians. Of particular relevance are articles 1, 3, 21, 24.1, and 24.2, which detail relevant rights of Indigenous Peoples with respect to human rights law, self-determination, the right to the improvement of health conditions, the right to traditional medicines and access to all social and health services, and the equal right to the enjoyment of the highest attainable standard of physical and mental health. For the full declaration, see https://www.un.org/esa/socdev/unpfii/documents/DRIPS_en.pdf.
4. For more information about the Signature Area Initiative at the University of Alberta, see https://www.ualberta.ca/strategic-plan/institutional-priorities/signature-areas-initiative/index.html.
5. As orally presented by Maria Campbell at a lecture given at the Humanities Centre, at the University of Alberta, on April 6, 2017.

REFERENCES

Adams, E. 2019. "Promoting Health and Wellness through Language: International Day of the World's Indigenous People." First Nations Health Authority. https://www.fnha.ca/about/news-and-events/news/promoting-health-and-wellness-through-language-international-day-of-the-worlds-indigenous-people.

Adelson, N. 2005. "The Embodiment of Inequity: Health Disparities in Aboriginal Canada." *Canadian Journal of Public Health* 96, Suppl. 2: S45–S61. https://doi.org/10.1007/BF03403702.

Asch, M., J. Borrows, and J. Tully, eds. 2018. *Resurgence and Reconciliation: Indigenous-Settler Relations and Earth Teachings.* Toronto: University of Toronto Press.

Banerji, A. 2020. "Urgent Resources for COVID-19 in Indigenous Communities." Change.org. https://www.change.org/p/prime-minister-trudeau-more-resources-for-covid-19-for-indigenous-communities-urgently-needed.

Belanger, Y.D., and P.W. Lackenbauer. 2014. *Blockades or Breakthroughs? Aboriginal Peoples Confront the Canadian State.* Montreal: McGill-Queen's University Press.

Big-Canoe, K., and C.A.M. Richmond. 2014. "Anishinabe Youth Perceptions about Community Health: Toward Environmental Repossession." *Health & Place* 26: 127–35. https://doi.org/10.1016/j.healthplace.2013.12.013.

Bombay, A., K. Matheson, and H. Anisman. 2009. "Intergenerational Trauma: Convergence of Multiple Processes among First Nations Peoples in Canada." *International Journal of Indigenous Health* 5, no. 3: 6–47.

Bombay, A., K. Matheson, and H. Anisman. 2014. "The Intergenerational Effects of Indian Residential Schools: Implications for the Concept of Historical Trauma." *Transcultural Psychiatry* 51, no. 3: 320–38. https://www.ncbi.nlm.nih.gov/pmc/articles/PMC4232330/.

Brown, S.M., C.N. Baker, and P. Wilcox. 2012. "Risking Connection Trauma Training: A Pathway toward Trauma-Informed Care in Child Congregate Care Settings." *Psychological Trauma: Theory, Research, Practice, and Policy* 4: 507–15.

Chandler, M.J., and C. Lalonde. 1998. "Cultural Continuity as a Hedge against Suicide in Canada's First Nations." *Transcultural Psychiatry* 35, no. 2: 191–219. https://doi.org/10.1177/136346159803500202.

Chandler, M.J., and C. Lalonde. 2003. "Cultural Continuity as a Protective Factor against Suicide in First Nations Youth." *Horizons—A Special Issue on Aboriginal Youth, Hope or Heartbreak: Aboriginal Youth and Canada's Future* 10, no. 1: 68–72.

Elias, B., J. Mignone, M. Hall, S.P. Hong, L. Hart, and J. Sareen. 2012. "Trauma and Suicide Behaviour Histories among a Canadian Indigenous Population: An Empirical Exploration of the Potential Role of Canada's Residential School System." *Social Science and Medicine* 74, no. 10: 1560–69. https://doi.org/10.1016/j.socscimed.2012.01.026.

Geddes, G. 2017. *Medicine Unbundled: A Journey through the Minefields of Indigenous Health Care.* Victoria, BC: Heritage House.

Greenwood, M., S. de Leeuw, N.M. Lindsay, and C. Reading. 2015. *Determinants of Indigenous Peoples' Health in Canada: Beyond the Social.* Toronto: Canadian Scholars' Press.

Guindon, F., with the Neeposh family. 2015. "Technology, Material Culture and the Well-Being of Aboriginal Peoples of Canada." *Journal of Material Culture* 15, no. 1: 77–97. https://doi.org/10.1177/1359183514566415.

Houle, N. 2017. "Improving Indigenous Maternity Care by Improving Access to Traditional Birth Practices." *birth issues* 30, no. 4: 43–45. https://bcaafc.com/wp-content/uploads/2020/01/3.-Houle-Improving-Indigenous-maternity-care.pdf.

Integrative Health Institute. 2017. "Proposal for Signature Area." University of Alberta. Unpublished.

Johnson, L.M., ed. 2019. *Wisdom Engaged: Traditional Knowledge for Northern Community Well-Being.* Edmonton: Polynya Press.

King, M., A. Smith, and M. Gracey. 2009. "Indigenous Health Part 2: The Underlying Causes of the Health Gap." *Lancet* 374, no. 9683: 76–85. https://doi.org/10.1016/ S0140-6736(09)60827-8.

Kirmayer, L.J., and G.G. Valaskakis. 2009. *Healing Traditions: The Mental Health of Aboriginal Peoples in Canada.* Vancouver: UBC Press.

Lambden J., O. Receveur, J. Marshall, and H.V. Kuhnlein. 2006. "Traditional and Market Food Access in Arctic Canada Is Affected by Economic Factors." *International Journal of Circumpolar Health* 65, no. 4: 331–40. https://doi.org/10.3402/ijch.v65i4.18117.

Littlechild, W. 2017. Plenary talk presented at the Integrative Health Institute Conference, University of Alberta, Edmonton, AB, October 27.

Marsh, T.N., D. Coholic, S. Cote-Meek, and L.M. Najavits. 2015a. "Blending Aboriginal and Western Healing Methods to Treat Intergenerational Trauma with Substance Use Disorder in Aboriginal Peoples Who Live in Northeastern Ontario, Canada." *Harm Reduction Journal* 12, no. 1: 1–12. https://doi.org/10.1186/s12954-015-0046-1.

Marsh, T.N., S. Cote-Meek, P. Toulouse, L.M. Najavits, and N.L. Young. 2015b. "The Application of Two-Eyed Seeing Decolonizing Methodology in Qualitative and Quantitative Research for the Treatment of Intergenerational Trauma and Substance Use Disorders." *International Journal of Qualitative Methods* 14, no. 5: 1–13. https://doi. org/10.1177/1609406915618046.

McDonald, L. 2019. "Encouraging Use of Conversational Kaska in Adult Speakers through Kaska Language Practice Sessions." MA thesis, Simon Fraser University.

Napoleon V. 2013. "Thinking about Indigenous Legal Orders." In *Dialogues on Human Rights and Legal Pluralism,* edited by R. Provost and C. Sheppard, 229–45. Dordrecht, Netherlands: Springer.

National Aboriginal Council of Midwives. 2016. *The Landscape of Midwifery Care for Aboriginal Communities in Canada: A Discussion Paper to Support Culturally Safe Midwifery Services for Aboriginal Families.* https://canadianmidwives.org/wp-content/uploads/2017/03/NACM_LandscapeReport_2016_REV_July18_LOW.pdf.

National Collaborating Centre for Aboriginal Health (NCCAH). 2016. *Culture and Language as Social Determinants of First Nations, Inuit and Métis Health.* https://www.ccnsa-nccah.ca/docs/determinants/FS-CultureLanguage-SDOH-FNMI-EN.pdf.

Oster, R.T., A. Grier, R. Lightning, M.J. Mayan, and E.L. Toth. 2014. "Cultural Continuity, Traditional Indigenous Language, and Diabetes in Alberta First Nations: A Mixed

Methods Study." *International Journal for Equity in Health* 13: 92. https://doi. org/10.1186/s12939-014-0092-4.

Reading, C., and F. Wien. 2009. *Health Inequalities and Social Determinants of Aboriginal People's Health.* Prince George, BC: National Collaborating Centre for Aboriginal Health.

Richmond, C.A.M., and N.A. Ross. 2009. "The Determinants of First Nation and Inuit Health: A Critical Population Health Approach." *Health and Place* 15, no. 2: 403–11. https://doi. org/10.1016/j.healthplace.2008.07.004.

Royal Commission on Aboriginal Peoples (RCAP). 1991. *Choosing Life: Special Report on Suicide among Aboriginal People.* Ottawa: RCAP.

Shield, D., and C. Martell. 2020. "RCMP 'Had No Understanding' of Sun Dance Ceremony That Was Interrupted, Dancer Says." *CBC News.* https://www.cbc.ca/news/canada/ saskatoon/beardys-okemasis-sun-dance-1.5566551.

Stewart, S., and A. Mashford-Pringle. 2019. "Moving and Enhancing System Change." *International Journal of Indigenous Health* 14, no. 1: 4–5. https://doi.org/10.32799/ijih. v14i1.32726.

Teegee, T. 2015. "Take Care of the Land and the Land Will Take Care of You." In *Determinants of Indigenous Peoples' Health in Canada: Beyond the Social,* edited by M. Greenwood, S. de Leeuw, N.M. Lindsay, and C. Reading, 120–33. Toronto: Canadian Scholars' Press.

Treaty No. 6. 1876. https://www.rcaanc-cirnac.gc.ca/eng/1100100028710/1581292569426.

Truth and Reconciliation Commission (TRC). 2015a. *Honouring the Truth, Reconciling for the Future: Summary of the Final Report of the Truth and Reconciliation Commission of Canada.* https://ehprnh2mwo3.exactdn.com/wp-content/uploads/2021/01/Executive_ Summary_English_Web.pdf.

Truth and Reconciliation Commission (TRC). 2015b. *Truth and Reconciliation Commission of Canada: Calls to Action.* https://ehprnh2mwo3.exactdn.com/wp-content/ uploads/2021/01/Calls_to_Action_English2.pdf.

Victor, J., M. Shouting, C. DeGroot, L. Vonkeman, M. Brave, R. Hunt, and G. Woticky. 2019. "I'taamohkanoohsin (Everyone Comes Together): (Re)connecting Indigenous People Experiencing Homelessness and Addiction to Their Blackfoot Ways of Knowing." *International Journal of Indigenous Health* 14, no. 1: 42–59. https://doi.org/10.32799/ ijih.v14i1.31939.

World Health Organization (WHO). n.d. "Constitution." https://www.who.int/about/ governance/constitution.

Yaphe, S., F. Richer, and C. Martin. 2019. "Cultural Safety Training for Health Professionals Working with Indigenous Populations in Montreal, Québec." *International Journal of Indigenous Health* 14, no. 1: 60–84. https://doi.org/10.32799/ijih.v14i1.30861.

2 *Spiritual Pathway*
to Health and Balance

HARRY WATCHMAKER

This chapter is adapted from the transcript of a conversation Harry Watchmaker had with Leslie Main Johnson and Riva Benditt (recorded in Edmonton, Alberta, February 26, 2017). His intent was to give a presentation as if he had done so at the Wisdom Engaged: Traditional Knowledge for Northern Community Well-Being conference, held in February 2015. Harry, of Kehewin Cree Nation, is a well-known Cree ceremonialist who works extensively with residential school survivors across Alberta, and with the urban community of Boyle Street Community Services Co-op in Edmonton, among other groups. He was one of the Traditional Knowledge Keepers who attended the Healers' Gathering held in conjunction with the Wisdom Engaged conference. He had responsibilities in the opening and closing pipe Ceremonies for that event.

Good evening, people. I would like to share some of my teachings and stories in the past. And my name is Harry Watchmaker from Kehewin Cree Nation. And I'd like to talk about culture, traditional medicines, and Ceremonies.

Really, culture first. Our way of life, in the past our language was oral language, oral teachings. Everything is oral. When I was young I learned my language, my culture, and spiritual ways. There was only one culture for me, and one language. Language was spoken every day, in the evening. And in wintertime my grandfather used to share some of the legends. Only in wintertime we are allowed to share the legend stories, and usually we do a Protocol in order for us to hear these legends. And now that we lose a lot of these Traditional Knowledge Keepers, I would like to see our language written so that some of the teachings that we need young people to get to know can be written down. Mainly, I'm here to support this book and remind people about the past.

In the past, life was very different. In the past, there were a lot of animals, a lot of ducks, a lot of fish, a lot of trees. There was so much plenty. Good water. Less interference. That was the past. Now today, present time, it's different. Less trees, less animals, less wildlife. Now today the animals are homeless. The farmers, ranchers, without any Protocol, they cut trees. If only they could learn from us, Protocol. How to respect the natural law. And the Earth and the Heavens.

And earlier I talk about the past, less interference. And today we have— influenced beliefs. Other people, they follow their cultures. Other languages. That's good, we share. We get to know each other. God's cultures and language. And cultural churches that we use. Elders, they really support the churches in the past.

Going back to the past—more local Traditional Knowledge Keepers were utilized, they were more used in the community. As time goes, they pass on, and [there are] less Traditional Knowledge Keepers in our community. So we have to adopt Traditional Knowledge Keepers from other communities, other reserves to continue the teachings that we had at one time.

Now the most important things about communities are the Clans. The roots where each family member comes from. Like me—I come from the Sun Clan. My name is Watchmaker. It's supposed to be Sunmaker in Cree. But the Indian Agent didn't write it the way it's supposed to be. But at this time we just adopt Watchmaker as our second name.

And going back to the roots and the relatives. Everybody was related. Everybody knows how they're related. And everything was good. And they get to know their Grandfathers, Grandmothers, their Dads and Moms, brothers and

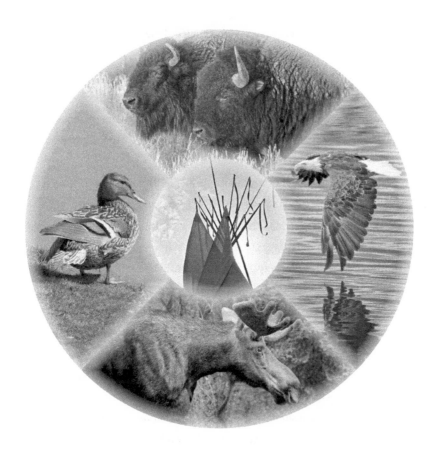

FIGURE 2.1A *Bison.*

[Photo by Douglas Bowen, licensed under Creative Commons 2.0. https://flic.kr/p/oX8cKu.]

FIGURE 2.1B *Eagle.*

[Photo by Erik Visser, used with permission.]

FIGURE 2.1C *Moose.*

[Photo by Erik Visser, used with permission.]

FIGURE 2.1D *Duck.*

[Photo by L.M. Johnson, used with permission.]

FIGURE 2.1E *Tipi at Truth and Reconciliation Commission hearings in Edmonton.*

[Photo by Riva Benditt, used with permission.]

sisters and family members, how they are related. Today it's the missing part of our life, how to relate to our youth and so on.

And also shelter is very important. Just for an example, tipis. Tipis were used in the past. Tipis are used today, for ceremonial purposes. And we call them *home fires*. Now those are today's modern homes. To keep these homes warm we need the Fire Spirit. And also in our vehicles, we need the Fire Spirit to keep us warm.

And the other important thing about the homes is the prayer. Elders used to sing every morning to greet the day. To help the young people to get to know the songs and to remind them they have a culture and language to hold on. What goes with the prayer is the smudge, cleanse ourself every day in the morning, and also at Ceremony. And also they usually smudge before we go to bed.

And stories were told by the Elders. They used to tell long stories, short stories. And the Legends were told in wintertime. These are natural law. Just follow the natural law. When to tell these stories.

Traditional Healing and medicines are part of our culture, and really, we get the medicines from Mother Earth. They start growing, start growing them in the spring. And then summer, and then fall we harvest the medicines. And also the food, and the smudge. And that's why Mother Earth is very important to us. Keeps us alive, and also keeps the animals alive—the birds, the fish, and so on. And the seasons are important. Spring, summer, fall, winter. Each season has its own spirits. And each month. It's very sacred. Like January is the Cold Month. And February, Month of the Eagle. Then March is Month of the Geese. April is the Month of Frog. And so on.

And also hunting is very important—trapping and fishing. I'll go to hunting first. Hunting is mainly in the fall. They hunt moose, deer, and so on. And wintertime and springtime they do the trapping.

And being healthy, each camp or community, it's very important. There they use the medicines they gather in the fall, and the Elders, and the Medicine Keepers, they keep all these medicines for the community.

And food, that was very important. Mainly we follow natural law. The moose, one of the basic foods of Native people and other peoples. It eats medicines. We have the moose, deer, and also beaver, rabbits, also, ducks, and so on.

And there's seven natural ways of healing. We do these every day. I'll just mention four of them.

One of them is *talk*. Talk is healing for everybody. That's communication. When you hear somebody talking, that's healing.

And the other one is *crying*. Crying is healing.

Also *music*, vibration. When you hear a drum or a musical instrument that makes you dance, that's healing.

And also *yawning*. The cat, the dog, the lion, they yawn. They prepare themselves. They're alert that day, so they're alert before something happens, they know what's happening. So all of us, we should practise yawning every day to alert our bodies for the day.

Now the Ceremonies. Mainly I'll talk about the basic ones. Sundance, Chicken Dance, Horse Dance, Ghost Dance, and Sweat Lodges, and so on.[1] They are very important in our communities. Mainly the Sundance. They prepare themselves all through the year. And the Sundance is usually in the summer months. Chicken Dance is all year around. Horse Dance, the summer season. Ghost Dance in the fall or springtime. Sweat Lodge, at one time it was only summertime. But now it's all year around. And it's very important to attend these Ceremonies, not only the people, they benefit from this, and also the animals, the birds, fish, they get life with the Ceremonies.

People from other parts of Canada they come to western Canada to come and learn our Sundance, or other Ceremonies. Now they find out these Ceremonies are the same as theirs, the songs. So they have a Sundance in the Maritimes. Alberta, Saskatchewan, Manitoba, and also in Germany, they have Sundance. They have powwows too.

OK, that's all I could say for now. Thank you.

1. For more on the contemporary importance of the Sundance Ceremony, see the *Windspeaker* article written by Jennifer Ashawasegai of Chisasibi (Ashawasegai 2012). For more on the Chicken Dance, also known as Pihewisimowin, or the Prairie Chicken Dance Ceremony, see Deiter (1999), which first appeared in Deiter-McArthur's collection, *Dances of the Northern Plains* (1987). For a description of the Horse Dance, see Ironstar (1993), and for a scholarly look at the Ghost Dance, see Kehoe (1968).

REFERENCES

Ashawasegai, J. 2012. "Sundance Is the Ceremony of Ceremonies." *Windspeaker* 30, no. 6: 18.

Deiter, P. 1999. "Men's Chicken Dance." *Saskatchewan Indian Powow* 29, no. 2: 14.

Deiter-McArthur, P., Saskatchewan Indian Cultural College, Federation of Saskatchewan Indian Nations. 1987. *Dances of the Northern Plains.* Saskatchewan Indian Cultural Centre.

Ironstar, M. 1993. "Horse Dance of the Plains Cree." *Saskatchewan Indian* 22, no. 1: 5.

Kehoe, A. 1968. "The Ghost Dance Religion in Saskatchewan, Canada." *Plains Anthropologist* 13, no. 42: 296–304. https://doi.org/10.1080/2052546.1968.11908509.

3 *Bringing Traditional Medicine into the Medical System*

CAMILLE (PABLO) RUSSELL AND

HAL EAGLETAIL

This chapter is based on a joint presentation by Camille (Pablo) Russell (Blood–Niitsítapi, Kainai) and Hal Eagletail (Tsuut'ina) at the Wisdom Engaged: Traditional Knowledge for Northern Community Well-Being conference, which took place in Edmonton, Alberta, in February 2015. Leslie Main Johnson transcribed the presentation. They are both healers based in Calgary, Alberta, and have worked extensively with local communities and with incarcerated persons. They focus here on their practice in collaboration with Alberta Health Services.

[Camille gives an introduction and prayer in Blackfoot before beginning his presentation.]

I'm very honoured to be here with each and every one of you today. I'm from the Blood Reserve, from the Blackfoot Confederacy from down south, and it's a great honour to pass the river into my relative the Cree's country here. And I'm very happy to meet all of you here, especially from the North. I've been here for the last couple of days and listening to everybody, and it seems like we have the same theme, wherever we come from. And we have the same problems, whether we come from the prairie or from the bush. And where I work, and I asked my brother here to help me out, he speaks better English than I do, and he's from the Tsuut'ina Nation, so he's related to you people from up north. I keep asking him questions like, "Is that your cousin? Is that your cousin?" "Yeah, that's my cousin over there." Yeah.

So I asked him to help me to talk, because we both work in the Alberta Health Services in Calgary as Traditional Wellness counsellors. So what our job is to go and talk. I work in a clinic and my brother works in the hospital, hospitals, and then we pray for the people. And then they come to the clinic and they ask to see the doctor, but they also ask to see me too. And I smudge with them, and I pray with them, and I give them some medicine. Sometimes, the doctor ask me, "He got better, what'd you give him?" And I don't want to tell him. I just say, "I just prayed for him," you know.

I'm scared to, so scared for the Natives to take our medicine and to use it, and we get nothing from it, you know. And it's time that for us Native people that we get credit for our medicines. For it to be protected. So it's not manipulated or taken from us. And I think it's important, we got so many medicines to help our people that it should start to be recognized by Canada.

But also, not just to be recognized, but to be protected, for us. So it's not—what's the word—exploited. And that we start to benefit from these things. You know sometimes the doctors, they give up on a patient, and then the patient goes and sees the Medicine Man and he gets better, and then the doctor wants to know, "What did he give you, what did he give you?" you know. We've got strong medicines. But we have to protect them. And I think that it's good that we work together, to protect, to protect everything. You know, we have to remember, and we have to learn from our Grandfathers. In their time, they didn't help each other. And if they helped each other, it will be different today. You know, today won't be the way it is today. So we should learn from them, and help each other, you know.

I have three teachers that taught me about herbs. Two were my two Grandmothers, and my Sundance leader. Three different teachers to teach me herbs. And they said to me, you know, before you can heal somebody, or help somebody, you have to heal yourself first. You have to be healthy first, before you can help somebody else.

So it took me a long time with my teacher, going around with him, before he start to tell me to talk. Because he was waiting for me to heal, from my pain. From my parents went to boarding school, and all of this. But I was raised with my Grandmother and my Grandfather, they didn't go to boarding school. You know, my Grandfather, his dad became blind, so he had to work. So he didn't go to school, and my Grandmother didn't go to school, and they had Dad when they're in their fifties, so they're very old people. And they're the ones that taught me many things, you know.

And so I just want everybody to touch your hair. That's the grass on the ground. Everybody touch your bone [rubbing wrist]. That's the mountains. Those are the rocks. Everybody look at your veins. That's the rivers. Everybody feel your breath. Do you need to brush your teeth? [Laughter.] That's the wind... that's the wind. And everybody touch your heart. That's the middle of the earth.

When you look at the river bottom or the mountains, you look at a deer or fox, they're beautiful. And when I look in this room, I see beauty too. When they say Mother Earth, this is what they mean. We are made in the image of our Mother. But our soul, that comes from the Sun, from the Creator. And the combination makes us a person, you know. And this body will have to go back to Mother Earth someday. And that spirit will go home where we come from. Where our ancestors go, that's where we go too, you know, someday. And, you know, in order for us to help each other, we first have to heal so we don't have jealousy. And competition. You know. We need to heal and love ourself, so we can work together. And help each other, you know.

And so this is what we do in Calgary, you know, we start to—people come and they ask for help and we use our herbs and our smudge and our songs, and we help them out, you know. And we—I never do something I do not know how to do. I know my boundaries because, the one my Gramma tell me that I have to answer to is the Sun. He is the one that watches me all day. And at night, it's the Moon. So I never overstep my boundaries, and if I don't know something, I tell people, "I don't know. But I'll get some help for you. I'll get the answer for you. And I wanted to share a song, but before that I would like my brother to talk a little bit more about what we're trying to do in Calgary, trying to make our medicines come together with the hospitals and stuff.

[Hal introduces himself.]

Tân'si, konnichiwa, bonjour, how...[Laughter; Hal gives more greetings in various languages.]

Does anyone have running water? Raise your hand. If anyone has running water, can you send her home, that's my wife! Ah, just teasing.

So really what, what our role is, it started here in Edmonton, the Traditional Wellness counselling, and it started here twenty years ago with Mr. Cardinal that spearheaded the first cultural helpers in the hospitals here. And twenty years ago, before that, we weren't allowed to bring medicine in the hospitals, the doctors shunned it, it wasn't allowed, it wasn't accepted, it was frowned upon. But Edmonton started to make movement. And we're very grateful for having this happen. And now it's been twenty years, just last year we celebrated twenty years, November, of having the first cultural helpers.

So now it's the norm. Now if you go in the hospital, they have designated smudge areas for us. We can have Ceremony in the chapels and bring in the medicines and the families can bring in their support as well that they're comfortable with, and one of the things that we still see as some barriers is the lack of opportunity to educate more. And educate the staff on how to have humble respect for the First Nation Aboriginal People.

And good-minded doctors that I've noticed already are the ones that can differentiate, just by last names, they can know a Cree from a Blackfoot from a Nakota. They also have understanding of the physical makeup. And those are the ones that really take an interest. That's something that we need to teach right at the university level. You know, this is a curriculum that should be a part of the doctors coming up the ranks in the future. The medicines that have been talked about here and the amount of exploitation that occurs and the billions of dollars worldwide, you know, that's the reason that our cancer Medicine People are scared to share. You know, they'll help people, they'll doctor people, they'll cure cancer. But they don't want to share because of that exploitation. And that's something that before I leave Alberta Health Services I'd like to see something in place. I'd like to see our pharmacies, our own health care centres, our own hospitals. You walk down Chinatown you can see the culture and the Chinese medicine being practised, adopted, you know.

Maybe in twenty years from now, we can walk down and go into a traditional herb shop, Aboriginal doctoring can take place for you there.

But people need to realize, we have to pay for these services. And when we talk to the old people, they give us examples of a pay structure. Chris from Australia, I really enjoyed your presentation yesterday.[1] Because you talk about there's a dollar value. And we need to start looking at these dollar values, because in the past, the dollar value was horses, blankets, robes. And you put that dollar value in today's terms, you're looking at ten, twenty, thirty thousand dollars. We need to start paying these spiritual leaders for their knowledge, and we need to recognize them.

So this is something that me and Pablo have been really pondering, how can we bring it forward. And thank goodness Alberta has a Wisdom Council. And we have some of the members here—the Nakota member Paul Daniels is here, he's a Sundance maker, and he sits on the Wisdom Council. And the Wisdom Council is an Alberta Health Service initiative. They have the ear of the CEO.

And Dr. Mustas has been part of all of that process. Give us a wave, doctor. Thank you. We also have one of the Wisdom co-chairs here, Mr. Rob Campre. Rob, give us a wave up there, Rob.

So, because they have the ear of the CEO, these are areas where we could bring forward some of these objectives. We hear a lot of things that happen with our people in the system. Well, this Wisdom Council can be approached and they can pass that on to the CEO. And it consists of Native doctors and nurses, but also Native Medicine People, Sundance makers, Bundle carriers, and medicine herbologists together, working together. And it crosses Aboriginal—you know, the Métis, the Inuit, and the Native. So that's the government word of Aboriginal, you know, they encompass all these three groups. And that's what is presented on this council, male and female. But I always have my doubts on government, there's always a hidden agenda because the word "Aboriginal," all the letters to the word "bingo" are in there. [Laughter.]

I know Russell, Camille, Pablo, it's part of his culture, his humbleness, not to brag of himself, or not to, you know make himself sound—you know, he's got to live a humble life. So I want to brag for him. He just came out with his own book.[2] Now this has only been a couple of months now it's come off the presses. And it talks about the Medicine Wheel teachings that the Blackfoot philosophy has reflected. It's really good for youth, teenagers, young people. But it also talks about the Medicine Wheel in all aspects of our lives, whether it's our work, whether it's corporation, whether it's community development, you apply this Medicine Wheel teachings to anything that you do in your life. And he's got them on sale here. He'll be selling them in the foyer. He'll also probably sign them, and maybe, maybe give you his phone number. [Laughter.] But I wanted to brag for him, because it's a really good book, and it's brand new, hot off the press.

I guess, just in conclusion for myself, our healers, we would be lost without them. And our healers are not necessarily the Elder age category now. It's coming down the ranks. You know, we have young spiritual leaders. And the term I always use is spiritual people, because we don't know how old they are. Some are gifted, some are twelve-, thirteen-year-old miracle workers. And they're gifted people. So I always make reference to spiritual leaders. But this one spiritual man, he came into the community, and he was healing the people. He healed a gentleman. Three brothers came in and one brother, he had a real sore back problems, and kind of slouched over. And that healer started to do his work on him, and next thing he's standing right up, walking, jumping around, healed. And the other gentleman, he had some diabetes issues, and that healer gave him medicine, and his diabetes was gone, and he was about to touch the third brother, and he says, "Don't touch me! I'm collecting workers' comp!" [Laughter.]

Anyways, we're gonna conclude with the Blessing Song. And one thing that Camille wanted me to mention is the new society that I'm starting, it's called the Sobriety Society. It's earning our headdress through sobriety. And to dedicate this, I shaved my head this past summer. I actually had one of the gentlemen running for the premiership of Alberta, Alderman Ric McIver, or Honourable Ric McIver, Minister, shave my head for me at our powwow. And the reason why I did this is because, you know, we always have the abuses that take place in our community, and our young people. And I always say, we have to find balance. It's not about "Quit this, don't do this, don't do that!" just, it's about balancing. So the society is really to earn your headdress. One feather represents four months of sobriety. And if you were to quit cold turkey, it'll be over seven years to earn your headdress, as part of the society. And being a part of a society involves certain rules, and respect and humbleness of yourself. And it applied to all ages, and to male and female. And that's something I'm just kick-starting now, and it's just in its infancy stage, but uh, look for the website in the future, ah I don't know, something like that... [laughter]. So thank you for your time, and blessings to you all here. Finished...

[Camille]
Yeah, so I just wanted to end with a song. I just wanted to quickly tell you a story there. There was this old man and he was sick. And he went to the doctor and the doctor said, "There's nothing we can do for you, you're going to die." So he was in the truck with the old lady, and the old lady said, "Well, let's go see the Medicine Man, see what he says." So they went to see the Medicine Man and the Spirit said, "We can't do anything for him, he's going to die." So he said, "Well, I guess, there's nothing you can do for you, you're gonna die." So he was in bed and he was in a coma and he woke up, and when he woke up, he woke up smelling fry bread. And he could say, "Oh, my wife is making fry bread. The last thing I'm gonna do in this life is I'm going have some fry bread." So he fell out of the bed, and he crawled down the hallway, and he climbed along the wall. And there his wife was busy cooking the fry bread and there was a big pile in a bowl. And she was making fry bread, and he was, with his last energy, he was trying to grab one. And then she looked over and saw him and she hit his hand and said, "Hey, don't take those, those are for the funeral!" [Laughter.]

[Camille picks up his drum.] Well, I want to sing this song from down south where we come from, because we're prairie people, and we follow the buffalo. And the buffalo is the only animal that faces the storm. Because the storm will pass quicker. If you see horses and cows, their back is always to the storm, but when you see a buffalo, he's always facing it. That's why the front part is furry. And when it's really cold, long ago my Gramma used to tell me, when it was really, really cold, the Old Man will put on his blanket and he'll walk around the camp and he'll tell the people, "What examples are you to my children? You men, you go hunt. You women, you go get wood and water. What examples are you to my grandchildren?" So the men, they have to hunt. And it's so cold the knife sticks to the meat. And the women they have to get wood and water, and that night they got a lot of meat, a lot of wood, and a lot of water. They survive. And where we come from, it's chinook country, so the warm wind come, that's when they rest. But all the people, we follow the buffalo. And that's why, you know, he faces the storm, and that's my encouragement, and I'm gonna sing that song. We play it from Writing-on-Stone where I heard it on the hill there. To follow the buffalo. And to give you that. So you walk into the storms. And the storms I'm talking about are the ones we create for ourselves. That we walk into our storms, and we fix them and everything. So that's the song I wanted to share with you.

There was a friend of mine from Toronto, and she was looking at a picture of a buffalo, and she said, "This's a buffalo." And I said, "Yeah, that's a buffalo." She said, "You guys shave them?" [Laughter.] And I said, "Oh, yeah all summer, we're shaving them, you know. Then we have a contest, who's the fastest one." She believed me, eh? [Laughs.] But, uh, maybe not to record this song, I appreciate that. [Recording paused while Camille performs a song.]

So. He use this. [Tapping heart.] When you talk to people you use this. This tells the truth. This says, I'm sorry. This admits when you're wrong. This one shares. This one [tapping forehead] wants the easy way out. This one wants to blame other people. This one doesn't want to say sorry. Doesn't want to share. He said, use this [heart] when you talk to yourself and to other people. Use this [brain] when you do math and physics. And when you know the difference, then you grow up. He said lotta people don't grow up yet. And when you want to make a decision that'll never change, they have to shake hands. So this is what she used to tell me when I was a kid. And I grow up and I teach my grandkids the same thing, and my kids too. But I would ask you something for me. If you would do something for me, I would appreciate it. Would you do something for me? Every time you look in the mirror, say, "I love you." And you'll make me very happy. Thank you very much.

NOTES

1. Hal is referring here to the joint presentation given by Christopher Kavelin and John C.
    Hunter the previous evening, February 19, 2015, during the second day of the Wisdom
    Engaged conference (see Kavelin and Hunter 2015).

2. Hal is referring to *The Path of the Buffalo Medicine Wheel* (see Russell 2014).

REFERENCES

Kavelin, C., and J.C. Hunter. 2015. "*Yilalu wangaan barigal-under*: A Long Time Ago in
    the Creation Time." Presentation at the Wisdom Engaged: Traditional Knowledge for
    Northern Community Well-Being Conference, University of Alberta, Edmonton, AB,
    February 18–22.

Russell, C.P. 2014. *The Path of the Buffalo Medicine Wheel*. 3rd Edition. Trykteam,
    svendborg, Denmark: ETNA Edition.

4 The Traditional Indigenous Model of Health and Well-Being

How Can the Western Physician Work within This Paradigm?

DARLENE P. AUGER

This chapter is based on Darlene's presentation at the Wisdom Engaged: Traditional Knowledge for Northern Community Well-Being conference, which took place in Edmonton, Alberta, in February 2015. The video-recorded presentation was transcribed by Leslie Main Johnson, and the written version was edited by Darlene P. Auger for inclusion in this book.

Hello, tân'si.

My name is Darlene Auger and I'm from Wasbasca originally. I'm a mother of two, and recently my baby girl, who has just turned eighteen, just started university here. And she decided to go into naturopathic medicines because this is the closest, I guess, form of education that she felt akin to, that relates so much to our way of doctoring, of being with people and working with natural medicines. I want to acknowledge my late parents Matilda and Patrick Auger, who taught me everything I know. And my grandmother, Adeline Cardinal, who is still with us. She is ninety-eight years old. And my great-grandparents, Louis and Mary-Louise Cardinal, who were both Medicine People.

And I want to share a story with you before I begin my PowerPoint presentation. It is a story about my great-grandfather, Louis Cardinal. My oldest brother shared this story with us family members. He said that my great-grandfather used to take him out to the bush when he would go pick medicines. One time when they had gone out, he had asked my brother to stay back—quite a ways back—and wait for him there. And he walked on. My brother watched him walk for a little ways. Then he knelt down on the ground, and he had a pot with him, like a basket, and he placed it in front of him, and he prayed with his tobacco for a long, long time my brother said, as he watched him. And he waited, and he waited, and he waited. And he wondered when my great-grandfather was going to get up and, you know, actually go pick the medicines. And then he said suddenly he saw—I'm getting emotional, sorry—he saw the plant come into the pot. And then my great-grandfather gave thanks and left with the plant in his pot.

And so, when we talk about medicine, as relational, as our relative, as being part of us, as being spirit, that's what we're talking about. And it's that powerful way that our people were, that our doctors were, that they could call on that medicine that they needed for whatever illness needed to be healed. And that it would come to them. And give its life that way.

I wanted to start my presentation off with this Indigenous world view (see Figure 4.1). And I'm looking in the audience, and I'm seeing a lot of brown faces. I thought that I was coming here to present to non-Indigenous physicians that might not have this knowledge of our world view and our ways of being and doctoring. So a lot of this you're going to know. The way that I've learned how to look at the world is that above us we have the Sky Nation, we have the sun, we have the moon, we have the stars. And just below that we have the waters. And then we have the land—the plants and the animals—everything that lives upon our Mother Earth. And then there's us. If you notice, we, the people, are at the very bottom. We're not at the top. We don't control anything. We don't have power over any of those things above. In fact, we rely on all of those things to live. If you take away any one of those things, we cannot survive. But if you take away us, the people, everything will survive without us just fine, even better. So, coming from this world view, we understand our humble place. And we understand that everything above us is in relation to us and is our helper. That's the way I've been taught. Everything is our helper. The animals are our helpers. The plants are our helpers. And the

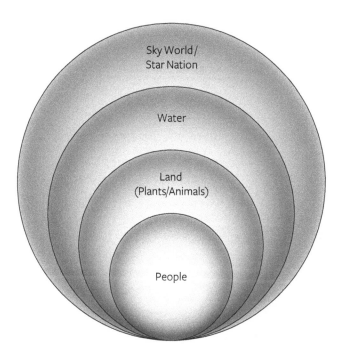

FIGURE 4.1 *Indigenous World View.*

water is our helper. Everything on Mother Earth is there to help us. It is not the other way around. We have no control over the land or anything above it.

This is something that's very common to us all, the Indigenous model of health (see Figure 4.2). In our Cree way of speaking, we call ourselves Nehiyawak. When we look at the morphology of this word, break it down, it actually means "four-part being," *Newo-lyiniw*. And the four parts of our being are the mental, physical, spiritual, and emotional. We believe that we came from a spiritual place, and we will go back to a spiritual place. As we live through every day, we live every single part of these beings. And in our body, our physical body, our spirit is able to thrive. And I found this quote, I thought it was so beautiful: "When 'I' is replaced by 'we,' even illness becomes wellness"—to cement the idea of relational well-being. Wellness equals harmony between all aspects of self and environment.

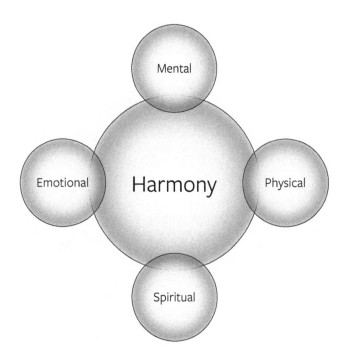

FIGURE 4.2 *Indigenous Model of Health.*

Earlier somebody talked about the longest journey that we will ever make in our lives—I think it was Pablo [Camille Russell]—the journey we make from our head to our heart. Our Elders talk about this quite often. In an article entitled "Balancing Head and Heart: The Importance of Relational Accountability in Community-University Partnerships," Kajner, Fletcher, and Makokis (2012) state,

> Very little happens without strong relationships. In an Indigenous world
> view, relationships require that partners self-reflect, and begin to decon-
> struct their own colonized understanding of self and other. It is difficult to
> grasp Indigenous approaches to research relationships when embedded in
> a westernized world view that emphasizes individualism. However, when
> non-Indigenous scholars engage Aboriginal people in heartfelt dialogue with
> patience and respect, the beginnings of an understanding are possible. This

understanding comes with a call to act: when scholars have engaged at the level of the heart, the responsibility for change sits equally on their shoulders. Understanding relationships in this way results in an ethical and moral obligation to become part of the movement for change. (260–61)

Ermine, Sinclair, and Browne (2005) captured this sentiment as follows:

Elders remind us to have "conversations" as equals. The act of dialogue is the act of resolving confrontation and is itself an ethical act. This will entail the examination of structures and systems in attempts to remove all vestiges of colonial and imperial forms of knowledge production and to instill respect and understanding of different and multiple readings, and different jurisdictions of the world. It will be in the ethical space where all assumptions, biases and misrepresentations about the "other" are brought to bear in the interests of identifying ethical, moral principles in cross-cultural interaction. (7)

It brings to mind one thing that often gets misinterpreted in our culture: the way that we allow our children to be. The way we just allow them to be by allowing them to make mistakes. We allow them to fall and learn from their mistakes. Often this gets misinterpreted as us not caring about our children. In our culture, we have an unspoken law, and it's the law of noninterference. Because again, we go back to that place where we *know* that—we are spirit, that we have our own journey here. And each and every one of us, including our children—they have their own journey, separate from us. And when we go into Ceremony, those children are not ours. They are the Creator's. And they become our siblings in that way. So this popular and catchy phrase—"the longest journey we will ever make in our lifetime is from our heart to our head"—speaks in part about this law. *If* we meet each other heart to heart, perhaps from that place we can begin to understand one another.

So I just wanted to capture some of our similarities and our differences in understanding self and the other:

Indigenous Medicine	Western Medicine
Four-part being (Newo-lyiniw)	Physical being
Home/land-based	Institutional
Relational	Individual
Natural medicine (land)	Pharmaceuticals (synthetic)
Spiritually based knowledge	Study-based knowledge
Personal	General
Subjective	Objective
Gifted and trained as a doctor	Trained and licensed as a doctor
Lifelong knowledge transfer (oral teachings)	Scholarly knowledge transfer (book learning)
Validated by community/people	Validated by a degree/institution
Compensated by gifts/honour	Compensated by money/wages

Places for health and well-being also differ:

Indigenous Medicine	Western Medicine
Sweat Lodge	Hospital
Home of doctor	Clinic

Should we be asking ourselves: Your way or mine? I think not. Somebody once said to me, when Western medicine stops trying to fit the Indigenous doctor into its model, perhaps we can begin to work together. But how can we do the same? Can we go and ask the Western physician to work within *our* Indigenous health model? What would this look like? Because in our world, a doctor is learning from a very early age, and it's a lifelong learning process of not only the craft, the disposition, and attitude but also the language and culture of the craft. Sometimes we come with a gift. We're born with that gift, of healing, of doctoring. So how would we bring the Western physician into our model of healing?

How do we move forward? Can we bring together the best of both worlds to create a new integrated health model? How? What would that look like?

What are the barriers we would face? What policies, beliefs, or systems are we willing to bend, change, or discard? What foundational support systems do we need to build? Are we willing to transform, brave, and act in order to create a path for our future doctors? These are some really hard questions that we must begin to dialogue about...perhaps we need to make that long journey from our heads to our hearts together. Thank you.

REFERENCES

Ermine, W., R. Sinclair, and M. Browne. 2005. *Kwayask itôtamowin: Indigenous Research Ethics*. Saskatoon, SK: Indigenous Peoples' Health Research Centre. https://ktpathways. ca/system/files/resources/2019-02/IPHRC_ACADRE_Ethics_Report_final.pdf.

Kajner, T., F. Fletcher, and P. Makokis. 2012. "Balancing Head and Heart: The Importance of Relational Accountability in Community-University Partnerships." *Innovative Higher Education* 37, no. 4: 257–70. https://doi.org/10.1007/s10755-011-9206-8.

5 The Healing Journey

Working for Kaska Wellness

MARY MAJE AND ANN MAJE RAIDER

Ann Maje Raider and Mary Maje are Kaska Elders. Ann was the first elected Chief of the Liard First Nation in 1992. After her tenure as Chief, she was active in the founding of the Liard Aboriginal Women's Society (LAWS) in 1998. Mary Maje is an Elder, land defender, and language expert from Ross River and also has been active in the Liard Aboriginal Women's Society since its founding. Both Ann and Mary are fluent in Kaska. LAWS has worked for Kaska wellbeing since the late 1990s, receiving funding from the Aboriginal Healing Foundation from 2001 until the program was closed, and held many activities at its camp on the shores of Frances Lake (Tu Cho Mene). This chapter is based on their joint presentation at the Wisdom Engaged: Traditional Knowledge for Northern Community Well-Being conference, which took place in Edmonton, Alberta, in February 2015. Leslie Main Johnson transcribed the presentation. Mary and Ann opened their presentation with a prayer. The chapter begins with Mary's contribution and ends with Ann's words, with a final comment by Mary.

Mary Maje—Introduction to Kaska Life and Land

My name is Mary Maje, and my Dene name in Kaska is called Atúd, because I was the youngest of all my family, so they call me "baby" in the language.

So there's five communities of Kaska people. We have a land mass of 96,600 square miles of land. They're all unceded territory, we did not sign any Treaty, no nothing. But we honour a lot of the people that know about traditional ways of living. I know many Tribes here have their own way of sharing their Traditional Knowledge. And we come from a matrilineal society where the woman is the teacher of our people. And the Land is, we have matrilineal land as well. So, when my son marries the opposite Clan, there is, we have two Clans, Nusgá Dena and Tsíyone Dene. So there's Wolf and Crow Clan. I'm the Crow Clan, and all my children are of the Crow Clan. My children would marry into the Wolf Clan, and my son, if he marries a Wolf Clan, he would move from my family use area to his mother-in-law's family, and he serve his wife's family for the rest of his life. So it's carried on like that.

Traditional medicines are kept very sacred among our people. We're not even allowed to run around on top of the plants. If we're going to pick traditional medicine, we ask God for it first. And we offer a gift before we can take that. And ask God to use that medicine so it could heal us. So, in those terms, and even the Dene, we have connections to the Land, the animals, the plant life—everything, we ask from God before we take it.

Dene á nizin—we're taught that from a very young age. It's the highest law of our land. We say, *Dene á nizin*. Means respect for everything. For all human beings, and we're never told "that is wrong" from our Elders. They always say, "You do it this way." If you make a mistake, they just tell you, "You do it this way." They never correct you. And there was nothing that's ever wrong, in a Dene sense. They hold us up—because all of us have that knowledge. Even a small child has the knowledge. They share the knowledge. So this is what we have learned from our ancestors.

So I'll just talk a little bit about our Kaska people, and I wanted to ask my sister to present more ways of our people. *Kula*. Thank you.

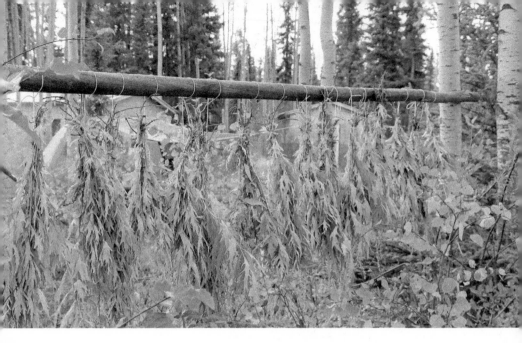

FIGURE 5.1 *Bunches of nón cho caribou leaves* (Artemesia tilesii*) hanging to dry at LAWS camp on the shores of Frances Lake (Tu Cho Mene), 2012.* [Photo by L.M. Johnson, used with permission.]

Ann Maje Raider—Activities and Programs of the Liard Aboriginal Women's Society

Good afternoon. My name is Ann Maje Raider. And I am currently the executive director and a residential health support worker with the Liard Aboriginal Women's Society in southeast Yukon in Watson Lake. Prior to that, I was the Chief of the Liard First Nations for six years in office, and after they elected a new Chief and council, I changed my direction. I came together with other Kaska women, and a beautiful project was birthed out of this painful change. We came together in 1998 and organized the Liard Aboriginal Women's Society. We offered a comprehensive healing project, which was funded by the Aboriginal Healing Foundation. This allowed us to build a camp at Frances Lake.

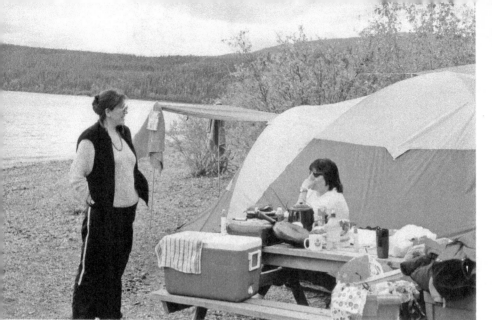

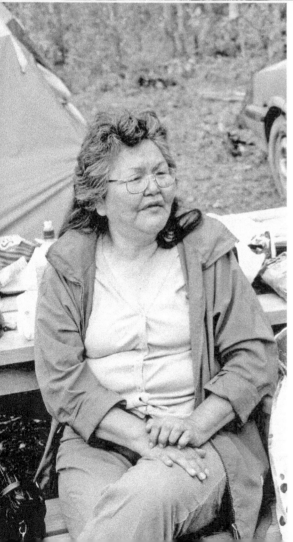

FIGURE 5.2 *(top)*
Ann Maje Raider (left) in
2000 at LAWS Camp on
Frances Lake (Tu Cho Mene).
[Photo by L.M. Johnson,
used with permission.]

FIGURE 5.3 *(left)*
Leda Jules at 2000 LAWS
Camp, Frances Lake
(Tu Cho Mene).
[Photo by L.M. Johnson,
used with permission.]

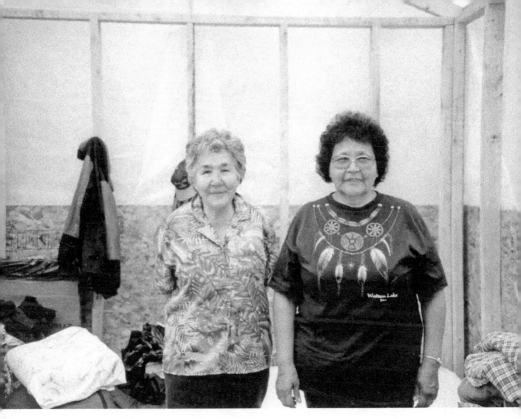

FIGURE 5.4 *May Brodhagen and Lorna Reid at LAWS camp,*
Frances Lake (Tu Cho Mene), 2000.
[Photo by L.M. Johnson, used with permission.]

We did many, many projects out there. They did tanning hides, they did
drying moose meat, drying meat for the winter, drying fish, picking berries, we
learned about our medicines, we learned how to can fish. We shared stories, lots
of stories, and there was lots of sharing. We lived there all summer, with the
Elders. And the Elders and people that were there said it brought back a sense
of belonging. We felt once again connected with each other. We were taking
care of each other, checking on each other, checking on the Elders, making
sure everyone had food. And what our old-timers like is to visit. I'm sure it's
like that in many of our communities. And that's what happened with Frances
Lake. We had time to visit each other. There's no computers or technology out
there, so it provided us time to really be with each other.

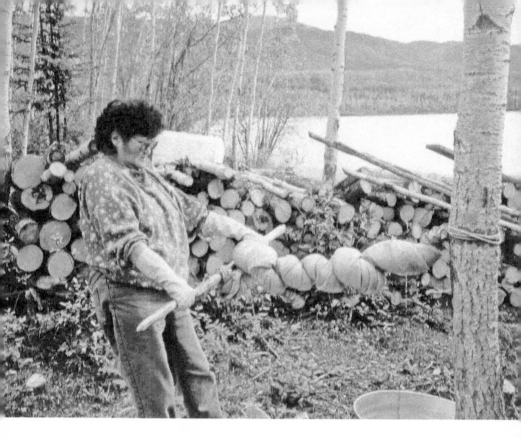

FIGURE 5.5 *Dorothy Smith working with moosehide, LAWS camp,*
Frances Lake (Tu Cho Mene), 2001.
[Photo by L.M. Johnson, used with permission.]

We also did a lot of Ceremony during that time—sweats, pipe Ceremonies.
I would every year for five years take our men down to Chilcotin, BC, and work
with a Traditional Healer down there. They would do traditional medicine,
Ceremonies, pipe Ceremonies to help them build their strength. We also did
peer support counselling with Dr. Alan Wade and Dr. Robin Routledge, who
are from Duncan, BC. And if you are interested in what they do, they do work
under a response-based approach to violence and understanding violence.
They take a response-based approach.

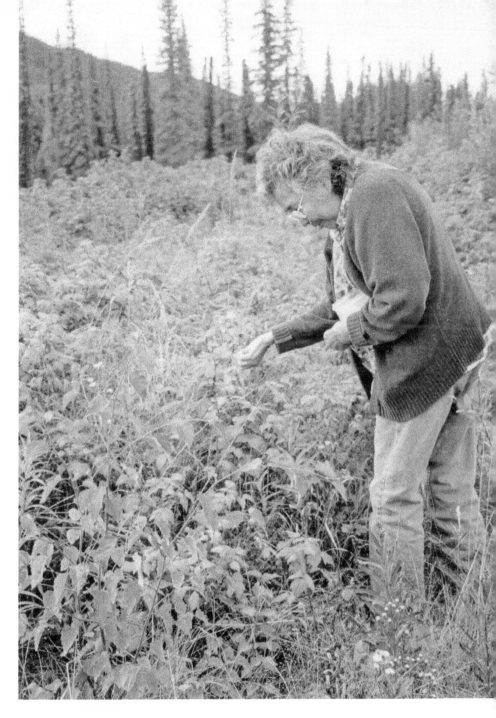

FIGURE 5.6 *Lorna Reid picking raspberries along Campbell Highway, 2001.*

[Photo by L.M. Johnson, used with permission.]

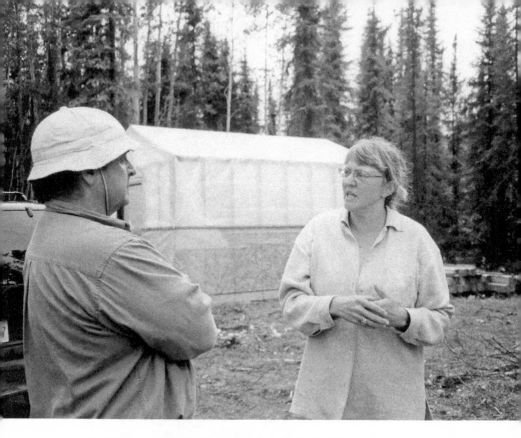

FIGURE 5.7 *Linda McDonald talking with Dr. Robin Routledge at LAWS camp, Frances Lake (Tu Cho Mene), 2000.*
[Photo by L.M. Johnson, used with permission.]

So, with the money from the Aboriginal Healing Foundation, we built our camp, and we would gather, hunt, fish, sew. We did everything, traditional. And we spoke our language. One thing we had a lot more out there than we do in the community is laughter. You would hear children laughing, and hear adults laughing, and it gave me a glimpse of what life must have been like prior to contact.

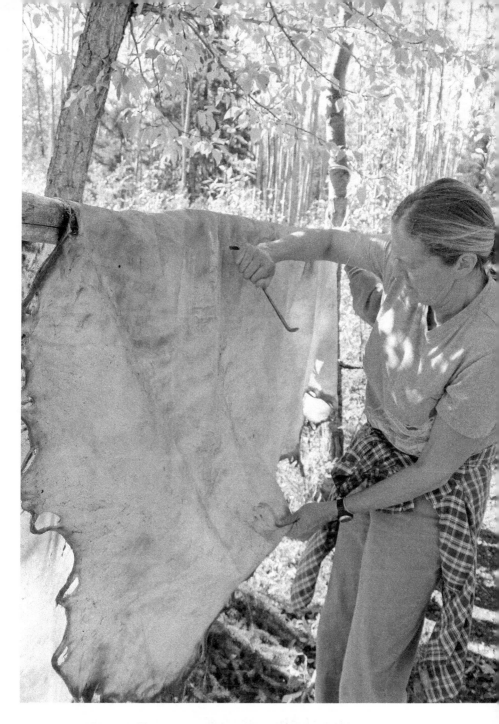

FIGURE 5.8 *Linda McDonald scraping moosehide, LAWS camp,*
Frances Lake (Tu Cho Mene), August 2012.

[*Photo by L.M. Johnson, used with permission.*]

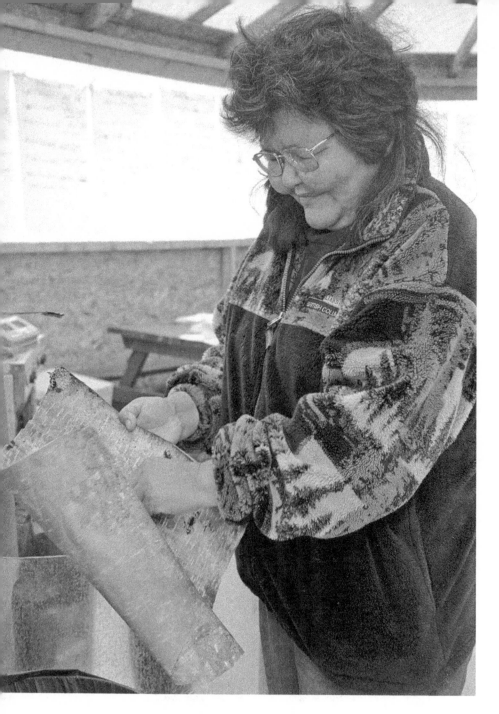

FIGURE 5.9 *Leda Jules learning to make a birchbark container at First Nations language course taught at LAWS camp at Frances Lake (Tu Cho Mene), 2002.* [Photo by L.M. Johnson, used with permission.]

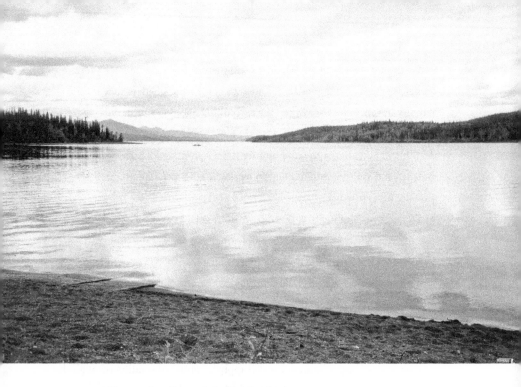

FIGURE 5.10 *View north up Frances Lake (Tu Cho Mene)*
from LAWS camp, summer 2000.
[*Photo by L.M. Johnson, used with permission.*]

Our connection to the Land is deeply spiritual. And I don't believe if you're a Dena that you can ever forget it. Because it's encoded in your genes. So you automatically have a connection with the Land. You would just have to go out and be in silence. Without all the gadgets, and you'll feel that. You'll feel that connection. And you'll hear your ancestors.

So, sadly, the Aboriginal Healing Foundation, as you all know, closed its doors. In 2010, we got funding from Health Canada. So Health Canada now provides us with a more limited budget. And what we do with that is provide residential health support workers. We provide cultural support, community cultural support. We have limited dollars to bring in healers, Traditional Healers. So we have brought in Robert Beaulieu.[1] He does one-on-one healing, and he's helped a lot of our people in our community through sweats and pipes and fire Ceremony.

We built the camp in 2000, and it's still there today. Originally, the tent frames were covered in plastic, but now we got them framed in, so we could actually use them for the winter. We're thinking of doing a proposal—there's a call out from Status of Women Canada for violence against women. I'm thinking of accessing it to build up a treatment program for men, to deal with violence and abusive men. If you can work with the men, then there is less violence against women.

We have no funding to run camp, we don't get a budget for camp and culture. When the Aboriginal Healing Foundation funded the project, it provided for funding for five Kaska communities to come in and join us. This kept all the people in Kaska communities connected. But now we haven't been together as Kaska people, so we're losing touch with our people down in Fort Ware [BC], because they're quite a ways from us, so now we don't get funding from the camp.

Because funding is limited, we also apply for proposal funding through the Anglican Church and the United Church. And they have funding that is there for traditional pursuits. It's limited, but it all helps. And then in the Yukon we have the arts fund from which we apply for funding.

We've done other great projects in our organization. We address violence against women, with Dr. Alan Wait. We work continually with him. And we've signed a Protocol with the RCMP. We did a two-year project with the RCMP and Dr. Alan Wait, helping them to understand violence and helping them to understand our culture, our people, and to not be so separated from us. That two-year period allowed us to develop a relationship with them. And at the first meeting, this is how they sat [stony-faced, arms folded across chest]. They sat across the table and all the Elders and women were on one side. They did not want to be there. But after—we always say we killed them with our kindness. Because we allowed the space for them. We weren't there to dig up old hash, saying, "You guys did this," or that. It wasn't about that. So we came together and signed a Protocol as to how we would work together. And currently the Whitehorse Coalition, which is a coalition of all the women's groups in the Yukon, is signing a Protocol with the RCMP that deals with how to create a better working relationship.

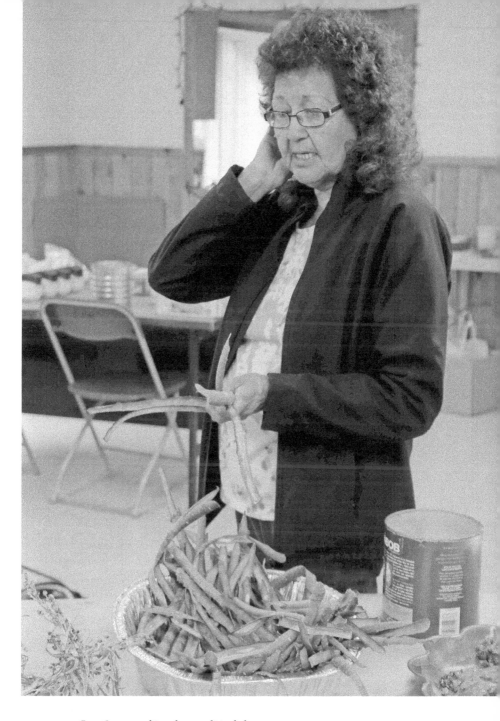

FIGURE 5.11 *Rose Caeser teaching about medicinal plants*
at community workshop at 2 Mile Watson Lake, summer 2015.
[*Photo by L.M. Johnson, used with permission.*]

We've done other projects with funding that we accessed. I want to say a slogan that I really like, which is "Nothing about us, without us"—to government. Because all too often government has developed policies and programs for our people which have only served to create harm, such as the residential schools. And we all know that government loves to research Indigenous people, or First Nations people. They like to put these great plans together and say how they're going to solve our problems. And dictate what will work in our communities. We come to the table, innocently, looking for solutions, having the solutions. But there's just no funding given to First Nations communities to do what we need to do, in a really big way, that's really going to create substantial changes. So, unless that happens, nothing's really going to change. Nothing in our community will be sustained. Because we keep going from one project to another project and nothing really gets rooted. These are the issues of insecure, unsustainable funding models. So, also, you're just looking for funding that's out there, so your whole mandate and what you do is driven by Outside.

In closing, I just want to say I witnessed the power of the Land and the nature of healing in the darkest places in many of our people. And it's so, so powerful. And during the Together for Justice project with the RCMP,[2] we went to the jail, and we asked our men there, you know, "What is it? How can we help? Tell us how you can help us." And they said, "We're really sick right now. We need help." And we said, "Well, how can that be done?" And they said, "We need traditional programs, we need to be on the Land. With programs with our Elders." And in the North, we've been asking for that, continually asking for that. And that funding door has not opened yet. But I'm very tenacious, and I don't give up very easily, so I always find another pot of money.

I believe the Land is very powerful. And it's healing because it doesn't judge us. It has no expectations of us. So nature is very healing because of that. And it provides us, it has provided us with centuries of food, medicine, healing, like at Frances Lake. Anything that we've wanted. We've been fighting, too, when I was in office, to keep industry out of that place. Because it's a very sacred place. And there's a lot of staking around Frances Lake for gold. So we have, like my sister said, we may have not surrendered our land, but the consequence of that is that you get so many outsiders in. The influx. The influx of taking up the Land, taking up that cultural land, taking up the sacred spaces. Because they're after the minerals.

We're pleased that in our Yukon and here that our ancestors and Elders are so, so connected to the Land and they're so rooted to it. I think part of that, too, is they're not so distracted with these things that go in your ears—Walkmans or text messages. So I'd like to thank you for your time today, for coming and listening to us and allowing us to share in our pictures of our great camp. We still do a lot, even though we don't have the money to go to camp as often we like. We do an annual retreat for the front-line workers at camp, and we bring in healers and people to take care of us for a week. So thank you. *Souga sin lá.*

Final Comments

Mary: Our people, they're so observant about the Land. The one Elder said he grew up around Frances Lake. And he said, "When I was a kid, that sun raise up right there" [gesturing]. "Every day when I was a kid," he said, "now the sun moved, it's over there, it comes up over there" [gesturing more to her right]. And his theory, he said, "It's the sun that moved. That's why there's all that things that are changing. That climate change has come. And that's even the leaves," he said, "if you look at it, it's really shiny, it's got oil on it. So, in the future," they said, "there's something going to go on the Land. There's something really clear going to run through that, something that's going to go all across the Land, that's where the fires will start." That's their observations. Thank you for that.

Ann: Thank you.

NOTES

1. Robert Beaulieu also attended and presented at the Wisdom Engaged conference in Edmonton, February 2015. His words are found in Chapter 17 of Johnson (2019).

2. For more on the Together for Justice program, a collaboration between LAWS and Watson Lake RCMP, see http://www.liardaboriginalwomen.ca/index.php/about-2/together-for-justice.

REFERENCES

Johnson, L.M., ed. 2019. *Wisdom Engaged: Traditional Knowledge for Northern Community Well-Being.* Edmonton: Polynya Press.

6 *Dim Wila Dil dils'm*
(*The Way We Live*)

Gitxsan Approaches to a Comprehensive Health Plan

RUBY E. MORGAN, LUU GISS YEE

Ruby E. Morgan, Luu Giss Yee, is a Gitxsan woman of the Gitwanga͟k Ganeda. She works to promote health among Gitxsan communities on the Laxyip (Territory). She engaged in projects related to holistic health planning and was instrumental in seeking funding from the First Nations Health Authority for a comprehensive health plan for the western Gitxsan. This chapter originated in a presentation at the Wisdom Engaged: Traditional Knowledge for Northern Community Well-Being confer-ence, which took place in Edmonton, Alberta, in February 2015. This written chapter evolved from that presentation to address the process of health planning, implementation, and ongoing events in northwest British Columbia.[1]

My grandfather was Ksuu, Ray Morgan. He was an Indian Residential School System (IRSS) survivor, a Second World War soldier, a carver, and a furniture maker. He worked for the BC Forest Service. He spoke as a profes-sional forester in the Delgamuukw trial. Following in his footsteps, I am Ruby E. Morgan, Luu Giss Yee, Gitwanga͟k Ganeda, Gitxsan/Celtic/German.

I present here Gitxsan approaches to a comprehensive health plan, the Gitxsan Traditional Health Plan. This is achieved by

- understanding *Dim Wila Dil dils'm* (the way we live),
- understanding *Wila da dils laxyip* (the way the land lives), and
- by all *sagyit ha'hle'alst* (working together).

Gitxsan health planning is based in supporting traditional values and community infrastructure by promoting preventative health care, realizing our assets as communities, and creating the capacity, in the spirit of truth and reconciliation, to return to the Laxyip (territories), a place of healing. We seek to be able to free ourselves from the "ghosts of residential schools" (Sim'oogit T'enimgyet, Dr. Art Mathews), so that we may be able to *Sip'xw hligetdin* (demonstrate the strength to speak in the Liliget[2]) once again as healthy Gitxsan communities.

We seek to be able to move beyond community members being held on reserves (effectively ghettos), moving beyond military-imposed (in the past and in the current example of the Unist'ot'en camp[3]) and current modern colonialisms (such as the Department of Indian Affairs, systemic under-funding of health and education systems), boundaries, and collective effects and trauma—the unfathomable depths of hatred and government corruption that have been unleashed upon our communities post-contact.

The planning undertaken thus far has helped us realize that effective execution of the plans for holistic community health requires a strong foundation in traditional values and language and the arts. This means embracing the individual's well-being, as well as the health of the land. Comprehensive health planning brings together all of these elements to create innovative traditional ways for promoting and improving community wellness on the Gitxsan Laxyip, and for emergency care at the Wilp Siipxw (Wrinch Memorial Hospital), thus addressing the barriers to healthy communities by using our assets: who we are as a Nation and the assets of the territories.

This chapter details the progress of our health planning and current initiatives to create land and Traditional Knowledge-based interventions and prevention by creating grassroots capacity building. We are acknowledging and promoting basic community rights in regard to safety and inclusion, as well as celebrating by remembering and supporting who we are. We work toward a renaissance of the Gitxsan Nation through the hereditary system, Matriarchs, the arts, language, and land-based healing.

Johnson (2019) detailed how Wrinch Memorial Hospital evolved during a transition stage from traditional community public health to institutionalized emergency care in the early 1900s. This hospital was supported by the Department of Indian Affairs, the Methodist Church (later the United Church of Canada), and the Province of British Columbia. Gitanmax Band gave the hospital twenty acres to build on. The Department of Indian Affairs provided a third of the capital to build the hospital in 1900, 1933, and 1977; in 1997, it donated ten million dollars (Kelm 1998, 136–37). It also provided more than half of the operating budget, since it paid for First Nations people to attend the hospital, reflecting the preponderance of Indigenous clientele: of the patients the hospital serves, approximately 85 per cent are First Nations (mostly Gitxsan and Wet'suwet'en), and 15 per cent are non-First Nations. The hospital has provided much-needed emergency care and should be included in the vision and direction of future public health planning.

Planning for Comprehensive Community Health

Seeking to identify, articulate, and support preventative health, based on Gitxsan traditional values by understanding Dim Wila Dil dils'm (the way we live).[4]

In 2011, we were provided with funding by the First Nations Health Authority[5] (FNHA) to create a Traditional Health Plan. We had five months and a very tiny budget to develop the Traditional Health Plan. Guidance was provided by Gitksen[6] Chiefs and Elders Tsu'alts, Amanda Zettergreen, and T'enimgyet, Dr. Art Mathews.

The Traditional Health Plan was developed in consultation with youth, Hereditary Chiefs, Band Council, Elders, interagency consultation, and consultation with the community at large, based upon the needs of the community. Consulting with the communities and presenting to entities as diverse as the Regional Aboriginal Health Improvement Committee, we organized gatherings on domestic violence and sexual abuse through End the Violence and local and national Indian Residential School healing projects and conferences.

We worked with Dr. Leslie Main Johnson (Athabasca University) and with other community leaders, Hereditary Chiefs, youth, and community members to realize the community's assets in preventative public health care. Therefore, now we are again on the forefront of preventive health care, creating a public health plan that all the community can use, including Band Councils, health clinics, the education system, youth, and Hereditary Chiefs. This plan has been added to the community planning and land use plans to make them even stronger documents. We facilitated two one-week workshops, created newsletters and posters, and arranged meetings to create an atmosphere of community unity and a common vision. Among the many meetings coordinated was a day-long meeting in Gitwangak with local, regional, provincial, and federal health representatives to discuss and support public health care in Gitwangak.

We established that we must centre our planning around bringing forward the communities' traditional Gitxsan hereditary social infrastructure, traditional language, the arts, and health care. Supporting these traditional structures ensures that traditional health governance is part of the planning process, along with economic development and education. Addressing issues of traditional food access, food security, and restoration of Gitxsan land management practices are also integral.

Language Defines Health Care and Our Health Care Practices

Language retention is vital to the health of a community, with research showing language is a significant predictor in reducing Indigenous youth suicide (Chandler and Lalonde 2008; Kirmayer, Tait, and Simpson 2009; Elias et al. 2012) and diabetes (Oster et al. 2014). Indigenous language learning was linked to impacts including achieving leadership positions within the community, healing from residential school trauma, and improved cultural and spiritual health.

As language defines Gitxsan health care, conversations around effective learning strategies, teaching methods, target demographics, and different strategies and policies are needed to help us understand how language defines our health care practice.

The Traditional Health Plan was added to the land use plan, changing it from a resource document to a document that reflects a Nation whose health is dependent upon the territories. This combination is more reflective of traditional Gitxsan land use management practices. (For more information, please see Leslie Main Johnson's "a tale of a trail" [2010].)

Rights to Health as Human Rights

We have come to a place where we are acknowledging what happened and are able to assess and redefine our health care system to reflect our strengths and support areas that need support. To thrive.

We get to tell our story. We get to dictate how the "health industry" integrates into our communities. We get to have long-term committed funding to support our Traditional Public Health Care Systems.

The United Nations Declaration on the Rights of Indigenous Peoples (UNDRIP) (2008) affirms the right to health as a human right, and it supports Indigenous self-determination with regard to health. According to UNDRIP, Article 23:

> Indigenous peoples have the right to determine and develop priorities and strategies for exercising their right to development. In particular, indigenous peoples have the right to be actively involved in developing and determining health, housing and other economic and social programmes affecting them and, as far as possible, to administer such programmes through their own institutions. (18)

In a similar vein, the Truth and Reconciliation Commission noted the importance of the right to self-determination. Seeking health is one dimension of addressing the ongoing impacts of colonialism. The principles that are to underpin this new relationship call for a recognition of Indigenous peoples' right to self-determination; constructive action on addressing the on-going legacies of colonialism; working towards a more equitable and inclusive society; respect for Indigenous knowledge systems and their guardians; "political will, joint leadership, trust building, accountability, and transparency; as well as a substantial investment of resources." (Truth and Reconciliation Commission 2015, 3–4)

In British Columbia, the First Nations Health Authority emphasizes the significance of cultural safety in health care:

Cultural safety in health care for Aboriginal peoples refers to practices rooted in a basic understanding of Aboriginal peoples' beliefs and history and a process of self-reflection regarding the power differential existing between provider and patient that may affect the process of care and healing. Cultural safety has been defined as a process of power redistribution that emphasizes providers' personal exploration of their own privilege and biases, and also as an outcome that is defined by the recipient of care and/or their family. (Dell et al. 2016, 301)

These declarations can only be fulfilled if all involved in the partnership are allowed to have defined practical expressions of their health care systems available. Gitxsan traditional community public health must be at the foundation of building these systems around cultural safety and humility. An example of this practical, cost-effective, community-based, prevention-based health care service is upheld and celebrated at the All Nations' Healing Hospital in Saskatchewan.[7]

Gitxsan on the Territories

Following the Traditional Healing systems as the determining structure, with a focus on maintaining good health naturally through the air we breathe, the water we drink, and the foods we consume, our daily physical movement and activities, rest and sleep, and interactions with other people is the way to achieve our goals of community health. It is how we live in our bodies on a daily basis; prevention is the overall Traditional Public Health Plan.

The Laxyip is imperative to the state health of all Gitxsan who live in the community and those that live away, as the hereditary system is responsible for all membership regardless of their location. Adding a Gitxsan Traditional Public Health Plan to the land use management plan thereby recognizes the Laxyip as integral to the protection and preservation of the Gitxsan Nation, which is essential to maintaining the identity, integrity, and well-being of all Gitxsan Wilp members.

As we are finding out through the overuse of resources, for the Laxyip to be used in ways that are unsustainable is an assault on the physical/dietary, mental health, and emotional and spiritual needs of the individual, family, and community, and would mean a deviation from the Gitxsan traditional holistic perspective.

Wila da dils laxyip (The Way the Land Lives)

Heal the Land—Heal the People
— DARLENE VEGH,
　　Gitxsan forestry and land use expert

Since time immemorial, the Gitxsan Nation has managed the territories through the development of complex social institutions, innovation, and land management. The Gitxsan Nation asserts Aboriginal title to and Aboriginal rights throughout its territory. We have long engaged and continue to engage in traditional activities throughout the territory now and into the future.

We have persevered. Many generations were devastated by colonization, the church, residential schools, and the intentional spread of diseases, actions now being acknowledged as a genocide. The removal of children blocked traditional grooming and transmission of knowledge. This trauma caused loss of identity and loss of self-esteem, affecting mental wellness, addictions and suicide, domestic violence, and disease.

Colonization was a destructive force that undermined the Gitxsan way of life and created a state of oppression so severe that to practice *Dim Wila Dil dils'm* (the way we live) would mean jail time or worse. Residential schools, the

Sixties Scoop, and now resource industry man-camp life prove that if you take the Gitxsan away from the Laxyip, the person, the family, and the community no longer have the necessary foundation from which to live a good, clean life.

> Matriarchs might not know their territory because they were away at residential school for so long...

> Youth have not been to the territory because of the generational effects of IRSS. Together we awaken and heal the territories.

Building capacity for Gitxsan in communities and on the territories is vital for healthy communities. This includes re-establishing traditional forms of navigation as people and land are reconnected. All such activities are based on multigenerational participation. The many generations of IRSS and the following intergenerational impact on our people, who have also been systematically disassociated with territory, language, and community, have created gaps. It is a planning priority to create spaces for Matriarchs and youth to come together on the territories—accessing the territories to overcome barriers to health and mental health.

> *The Gitxsan never get lost, they just run out of daylight.*
> — MENTOR SIM'OOGIT T'ENIMGYET, DR. ART MATHEWS

Below I discuss two programs that we are developing to support the implementation of the Traditional Health Plan—"knowing from the heart."[8] The first is Self-Regulation Therapy (Trauma Training www.cftre.com) training for Territorial Guides and community front line workers in the area of mental health. Planning for healing on the territories requires many steps. With the Self-Regulation Therapy training, people can gain access to the territories with someone safe and knowledgeable. For clients to be taken out on day trips, the Territorial Guide or Laxyip guide would be able to help support their healing process through the Self-Regulation Therapy training and working with the "team," which would include the therapist/wellness counsellor.

The second is the Introduction to Traditional Territorial Management Program. This includes contributing to traditional territorial knowledge by mapping their own territories, being able to access traditional systems, and being in contact with the Chief to ask for permission, report findings, and add collected data to the Territorial Atlas. Clients would also be taught about traditional resources and land-based knowledge as they worked. In this process, the client would also be taught GIS/GPS data collection skills; basic map, compass use, and navigation skills; traditional navigation by place name, not by the four cardinal directions (involving recovering language skills); and territorial life skills. Gitxsan life skills are based on remembering who you are in context, in relationship to community and territories. This gives you the ability to provide for yourself, family, and community.

Traditional Relationships

It is the Ceremony that invites the person to Heal.
— SIGIDIMHANA<u>K</u> WII SEE<u>K</u>S, BEVERLEY ANDERSON

This next section of the chapter shares words and perspectives from facilitators who came in to work with community members at the Tan Gisst Culture Camp, held on the Laxyip of Sim'oogit Guxsen in the summer of 2016. At this camp, the principles of the Gitxsan Traditional Health Plan were put into practice. Facilitators worked with community members to support healing, teach Gitxsan skills and art, and aid participants' learning about who they were, through being on the land.

Tam Gisst Culture Camp was established to create a healing space for people to feel safe and to be able to find resources from the territories and guidance through the hereditary system, as this is the Gitxsan prescription. The usual prescriptions for healing from the medical establishment are either not locally available, or are not applicable to the Gitxsan.

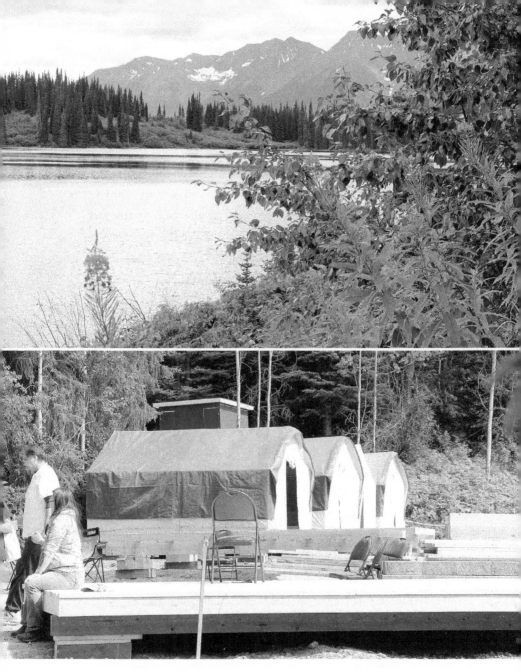

FIGURE 6.1 (top) Tam Gisst, the lake and setting for the camp, July 2016.
[Photo by L.M. Johnson, used with permission.]

FIGURE 6.2 (bottom) Tam Gisst camp, July 2016.
[Photo by L.M. Johnson, used with permission.]

Frank Shannon and Damian Abramson

They brought their drums and blankets.

Haida facilitators and mental health professionals Frank Shannon and Damian Abramson joined us at the camp to provide mental health supports. They immediately set everyone at ease by showing their knowledge and support of who we are as Gitxsan people:

The high quality of facilitators and camp staff allowed the dynamics to gel almost immediately. The amazing traditional/contemporary chefs not only completely understood the respect and teachings that go into feeding our people, but were a wealth of knowledge to staff and all participants.

The men got to experience true oral culture from a matriarchal[b] tribal system, with shared stories of their ancestry. By the second day as evidenced by the settling of all people's nervous system involved in the camp; that being on the territory was a larger-than-life resource and could not be measured in value. Being at the camp allowed Elders and facilitators to become more regulated which allowed the men the opportunity to be taught in the same manner as our ancestors. The teachings on the territory connected many of us to stories untold in the Western setting and the abundance of medicine in the territory also engaged them in their own stories. This opportunity to learn and knowledge share brought a sense of confidence and pride to the participants which also helped to regulate their nervous systems. It was amazing to witness the connection with despair as the conversation turned to intergenerational trauma and health and wellness struggle in our communities for the men. I then witnessed a natural shift to resource as the topic of food gathering was presented. It was an instant settling of our nervous systems as we spoke of gathering and preserving fish, the comparison of ocean and river fish, what species of fish was better to smoke, what trees taste best to smoke with, and how long to smoke. This was a connection to the past that reminded the men of the resilience passed on from their ancestors and remained a responsibility to pass on to the next generations.

*I feel the camp was overwhelming success due to strong visioning, coor-
dinating, support and funding from community, talented staff, professional
facilitators, respectful Elders, incredible chefs, courageous participants, and
mostly the healing the beautiful territory provided.*

— FRANK SHANNON, OODCADJAAWAA, EAGLE WHO HUNTS,
Eagle Clan

Virginia Morgan

Virginia is an artist, teacher, and change maker, and taught Gitxsan design
and art to participants. She wrote:

*When students learn out on the territory, they have a sense of belonging. They
learn to respect themselves, others that they are working with, and the land.
While learning on the land, they are able to reflect on the daily blessings,
obstacles, as well as on their own lives. Being out on the territories, out in
natural surroundings, youth are working as a team. They are working cooper-
atively, as a collective, working towards one goal. They learn what their roles
and responsibilities are while they are out there. Through daily discussions,
they also learn how these same roles and responsibilities can be transferred
over to their home life.*

*Being out on the land with a matriarch offers the youth an opportunity
to hear stories and their own adaawx, which is crucial for them to know the
history and laws of the Gitxsan. It is also important that they hear and begin
to recognize their own family history.*

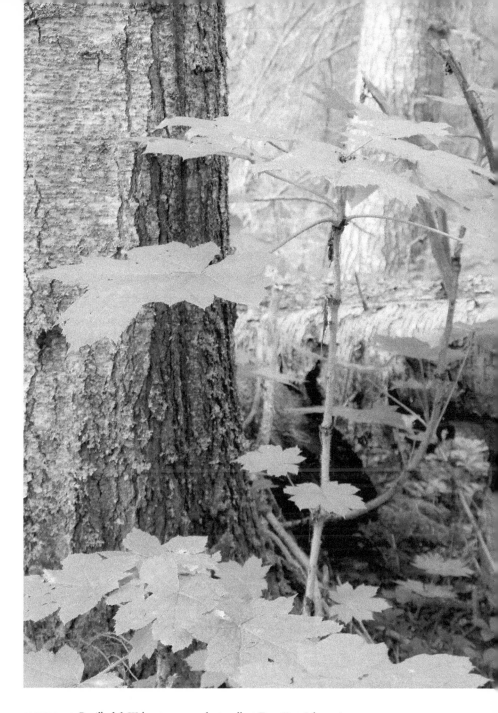

FIGURE 6.3 *Devil's club Wa'umst, seen on plant walk at Tam Gisst, July 2016.*
[*Photo by L.M. Johnson, used with permission.*]

Frances Jackson, Wii Au̲x̲, and Sylvia Johnson

Elders from Gitanmaax Frances Jackson, Wii Au̲x̲; and Sylvia Johnson, who have lived for many years in Prince Rupert and in Gitwanga̲k, came to share their skills.

We taught net mending (gillnets), where the participants learned how to prepare the equipment needed for mending as well as how to repair the net. Mending requires a tremendous amount of focus and manual dexterity. The repetitive motions and ability to see the flaws and inconsistencies within the work can translate across to recognizing opportunities as they arise, being aware of the impact of positive and negative communication, and creating an understanding of the patience and resilience that our everyday lives sometimes require.

We also taught traditional cedar harvesting and prepping. There are several steps needed to prepare cedar for weaving. The traditional harvesting speaks directly to our relationship to all things and our connection to the land. In taking only what the tree gives and ensuring that the tree will live through the process and after, shows a deep-seated respect that is given automatically. In harvesting as a group we moved through the forest sharing the traditional knowledge of the activity but also sharing our diverse backgrounds throughout the day. As is our culture we were very fortunate to share a meal out on the land and take the very important time to regenerate and reflect on the ideals and virtues that brought us all together in that place. Weaving, like mending, is another way for us to be in our place and in the moment. This is a gift that is very much taken for granted and overlooked in today's product based society. These are activities that speak to process, to ongoing learning, and to allowing something to become something rather than needing it to be something right now.

At the camp we were essentially off the grid with no electronic gadgets or cell service, so we had everyone's attention. Being out in the forest is very relaxing, the air is so clean, just the smoke from the campfire. We gathered around in the campfire in the evening with young and old actually conversing and reflecting on the events of the day and sharing memories that the day brought forth; and we laughed a lot.

— FRANCES JACKSON, WII AU̲X̲

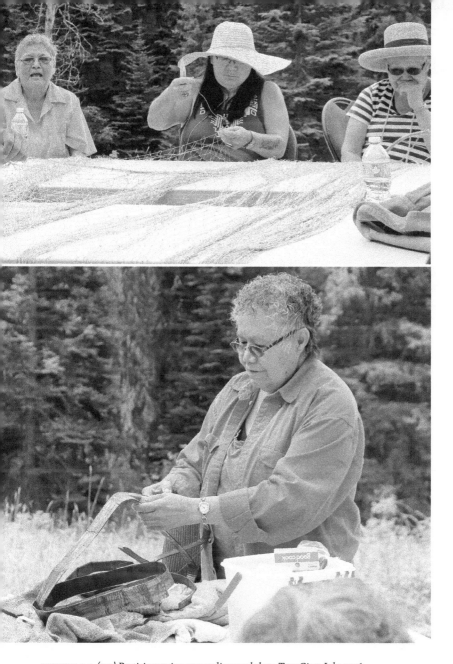

FIGURE 6.4 *(top) Participants in net-mending workshop, Tam Gisst, July 2016.*
[Photo by L.M. Johnson, used with permission.]

FIGURE 6.5 *(bottom) Frances Jackson, Wii Au̱x̱, teaching cedar bark weaving*
at the Tam Gisst camp, July 2016.
[Photo by L.M. Johnson, used with permission.]

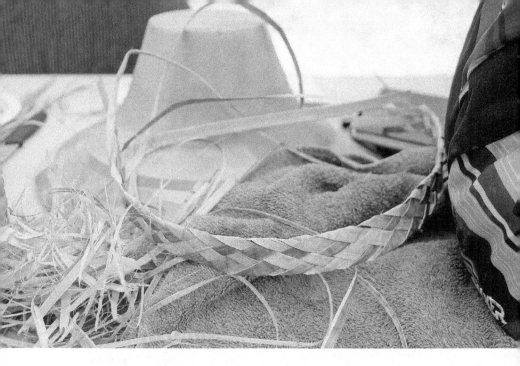

FIGURE 6.6 *Wooden hat form, and samples of cedar bark weaving,*
at Tam Gisst camp, July 2016.
[Photo by L.M. Johnson, used with permission.]

Culture camps have a great potential for healing. However, supports for clients when they return home may be challenging. There are many gaps in services for our communities, and funding budgets are always well below actual costs. Due to capacity limitations, service providers have a difficult, if not impossible, task of fulfilling mandates. There are healing/rehabilitation facilities in most major centres, and even one in our community. After clients return home from these facilities, even in our community with the healing centre/rehabilitation, there are few if any supports and/or activities. The healing/rehabilitation centre in our community does very little community outreach.

A key path forward is to recognize that a culture camp effectively serves as a trauma centre and is the way to recover from a cultural genocide. For the Gitxsan to be reconnected in a foundational way once again to the Laxyip would substantially improve the standard of life and state of health for the membership.

Establishing culture camps allows for traditional programming to address the following important areas:

- Depression
- Suicide
- Domestic violence
- Addictions
- Anger management
- Conflict resolution
- Pre/post-natal parenting
- Nutrition and food security—how to identify, harvest, and prepare traditional foods
- Elder care
- Self-care

This is only a progress report—we have found a way forward. We have found a way to free ourselves from the "ghosts of residential schools" (as mentor Sim'oogit T'enimgyet, Dr. Art Mathews, phrases it), so that we may be able to *Sip'xw hligetdin* (demonstrating the strength to speak in the Liliget) once again as healthy Gitxsan communities.

Reflections on Planning for Gitxsan Community Health
Planning for and with Galts'ep (Communities)

Wilnadehl (family) and *xaldawkxw* (medicine) are key concepts.

A different kind of education creates a different kind of consciousness.
— CASH AHENAKEW,
     Canada Research Chair in Indigenous Peoples' Well-being

Similarly, a different kind of healing creates a different kind of health consciousness. By supporting the Matriarchs within a Gitxsan Traditional Public Health Plan, we are not looking to replicate a health or educational institution. We are supporting a Gitxsan model of healing, health, and prevention in the individual, family, Clan, and community grounded in traditional community supports and land-based healing that promotes Gitxsan values and ethics. We have been advocating for this for the past thirty years, as this quote from the Gitxsan Health Society (1986, 1) reflects:

> It is the responsibility of the community as a whole to be healthy and the tendency for Gitxsan is to look at healing from traditional concepts.
>
> Families, wilp groups, clans, friends and neighbours provide much of the "front line help"; to their detriment this has gone unrecognized and unsupported by the "external systems" in place. The "external systems," rather than supporting and enhancing the ability of the family, clans, wilps and communities to care for their members, tend to take over and shift responsibility, ownership and control away from the community. Thus, an artificial division is created between the "natural community based systems" and the often "external punitive emergency systems."

By representing these traditional community structures, Gitxsan traditional public health empowers and supports community systems by supporting individuals and families in their homes for palliative and respite care, as an example.

For the most part, our families and communities take care of the elderly, disabled, and palliative care at home. We are not inclined to require facilities that would institutionalize our health care. Capital costs are saved, as huge facilities to house people are not needed. Employees live and work in the communities, so housing and safety can be addressed. Gitxsan communities and families are now asking that they be supported in the traditional way throughout the process. Traditional health care is preventive, and cost-effective health care is community-based. This is important, as Gitxsan traditional public health is being defined by the communities, the obvious barriers to hospital health care are removed. By two health care systems—the hospital and the First Nations communities—working together, we create positive, inclusive health care for all demographics.

It is important to support and fund improved primary and community care delivery. The ability of a laboratory in a hospital to be more cost-effective depends on strong home and community care programs ready to accommodate these discharged clients who may require results, further testing, and continuing care. At the All Nations' Healing Hospital, there is a direct connection to the communities, and this allows for quality and safety of health care that is cost-effective and supports traditional ethics and values.

Consultants and other experts continue to design health care around their image and biases. Sometimes they even use data and/or the absence of data to benefit from First Nations. When the "health area" maps are overlaid for service delivery, or consultants looking for funding opportunities, it seems that the reality of the demographic, geography, and First Nations' abilities to determine and implement a health care system are interfered with and their interests ignored. The dismal attempt at quality and safety of health care is unavoidable, because it is done out of context of who we are as a people for Gitxsan, Wet'suwet'en, and other First Nations. By using our Nations maps as the "service area," it seemingly, simply solves one barrier to "service delivery."

Traditional Gitxsan public health planning is the basis for health care within the Gitxsan territories, providing a healing process that is both traditional and holistic. Given that the Gitxsan traditional structures still remain and are valid, through the traditional consensus processes the community is given the opportunity to speak and be heard, and thereby a healing process for the entire community evolves. This serves not only to empower individuals and families, but communities, Wilps, and Clans are also taken into account in the holistic process. Most service models are intervention-oriented and do not follow the Gitxsan holistic vision of healing. Traditional public health planning allows the Gitxsan to initiate and support a health care system that is built upon the strengths and resources of the community. This in turn allows the community to fully benefit from outside services.

Gitxsan have been conducting, implementing, and doing the best practices in traditional public health since *Gwal yee* (time immemorial) that have been shown to be effective within our own communities. Gitxsan communities are going without services, treatment, and prevention programs, because the ones we would implement are ineligible for funding, while the ones that are recommended and delivered do not fit our community needs.

Culturally validated, which is very different than the integration of "First Nations culture," refers to those approaches that are based upon principles, laws, and values of Gitxsan communities. These *si wilayinsxw* (teachings) form the basis for practical public health planning. They are culturally relevant, culturally appropriate, and designed according to Gitxsan Traditional Public Health. Furthermore, they have been implemented according to the community's accepted practices and accepted as valid. They have also been evaluated and studied by many academics (e.g., Johnson 1997, 2006, 2010; Daly 2005; Marsden n.d., 2008). Their effectiveness has been demonstrated and defended.

Wilp Siipxw (Wrinch Memorial Hospital):
Challenges, Racism, and Equity

Bringing both medical systems together has yet to work. A Traditional Gitxsan Public Health Plan should be the basis for health care within the Gitxsan territories; outside health services should be integrated into this foundation. This Traditional Public Health Plan allows the Gitxsan to initiate and support a health plan that is built upon the strengths and resources of the community. One aspect of collaborative care is how to bring traditional community practices together with emergency medical and hospital care.

Wrinch Memorial Hospital is operated by the Northern Health Authority in Hazelton, British Columbia, Gitxsan Nation.[10] It provides acute, complex, and community care, assisted living, and short- and longer-term staff accommodation. Services include emergency, obstetrical and operating room services, lab, X-ray, ultrasound, dieticians, and occupational therapy.

In January 2012, Pauline Cole and Vernon Joseph, who both died while the case was still active, filed a class action suit with the BC Human Rights Tribunal on behalf of First Nations groups in the hospital's service area. In January 2016, the long-running human rights lawsuit that accused Wrinch Memorial Hospital administration of discriminating against First Nations people in the Hazelton area (Gitxsan and Wet'suwet'en territory) was settled out of court.

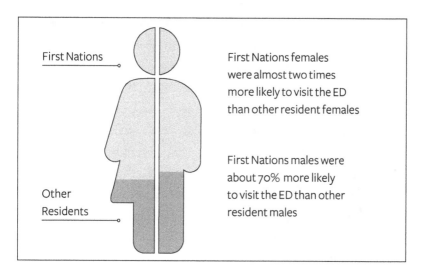

First Nations

First Nations females were almost two times more likely to visit the ED than other resident females

First Nations males were about 70% more likely to visit the ED than other resident males

Other Residents

FIGURE 6.7 *Use of emergency room services by Indigenous women and men. Redrawn from First Nations Health Authority (n.d., 5).*

Doctors, academics, policy makers, providers, consultants, and administration make most of the planning and decisions regarding our health care. Seemingly, so many interests are being represented—except those of patients and the community. This adds to the proven barriers of racism, stigmatism, and denied care as reported by the Humans Rights Tribunal. These types of interactions are still happening.

To respond to these concerns, the BC Human Rights Tribunal established the CHIC (Community Health Improvement Committee), a new independent community health group with a mandate to collaboratively co-design a solution to these concerns. The purpose of CHIC is to identify and close gaps in health outcomes for both Aboriginal and non-Aboriginal communities (*The Interior News* 2016, A-18).

Gitxsan Nations have raised concerns that their members utilize emergency department services at rates higher than non-Gitxsan Nation members (Figure 6.7), and that both patient experience and patient outcomes in many areas are relatively worse (CHIC n.d.a, n.d.b).

Gitxsan/Wet'suwet'en Traditional Public Health and Northern Health/ Wrinch Memorial, FNHA are integral yet distinct systems. All must work together to ensure continuity of care for our communities. The CHIC committee was put in place to change the paradigm of health care from one of inequities, racism, and associated higher health care costs. The time for fundamental health policy renewal to address these issues is long overdue. As an independent committee representing the communities, CHIC is well placed to lead these efforts.

By bringing local First Nations public health care through a health systems change based on traditional and community care, to uphold our rights to cultural safety and humility, we then create a template for other Nations to further define their traditional and community health, just as we have referenced the All Nations' Healing Hospital in Saskatchewan. With this visioning and planning in place, we are able to integrate other health care partners and service providers into our systems where their basic understanding of Aboriginal Peoples' beliefs and history has support and is relevant. By following this process, we can offer partners practical solutions that reflect the communities, research, data, demographics, and budgets.

Unfortunately, almost all of our doctors, nurses, and mental health professionals are non-First Nations. Typically, they do not have the required lived experience to support and work along with the community. Working with one another would require these professionals to immerse themselves into the Nation they are attempting to assist, learning the language and social infrastructure as they would if they attempted to work in any other country.

We are at an awkward moment, where our service providers and funders are perhaps realizing they have more in common with missionaries than with our communities and could possibly be doing just as much damage as the IRSS (Indian Residential School System) and Sixties Scoop.[11] Their bureaucratic positions are unable to build capacity to service our communities. They have mandates to provide mental health and other important health and education services, but not the budgets. How much funding will it take to heal a genocide? Although we have begun to educate and train, many health professionals do not stay very long, and we begin this education again with the new health professional a few months later. We had to take the government to court to prove our points,[12] and there are still no changes to address either the underfunding by one-quarter to one-third in health and education and the human rights issues at Wrinch Memorial Hospital.[13] In this huge crevasse of service gaps, people are dying, generations are dying. This Traditional Public Health Plan is the start of designing, developing, and delivering appropriate training and education programs based on Gitxsan concepts of health, illness, medicine, and treatment.[14] One example: outsiders easily misdiagnosed cultural experiences, such as visions and spiritual experiences, as serious psychological impairment requiring clinical treatment, when a traditional approach would address many of the healing requirements, understanding spiritual contexts, and holistic mind/body/spirit integration. Concern has also been expressed regarding the over-medication of Elders, and how this disrupts the traditional spiritual journey. A drugged mind or spirit may be unable to clearly perceive or receive spiritual guidance necessary to healing, or to the passage from this life.

According to the First Nations Health Authority (n.d.), First Nations had lower rates of use of physician services in 2014–2015 compared to other residents, including GPs seen outside of hospitals, medical specialists, surgeons, oncologists, and physical rehabilitation physicians. Their use of laboratory testing was also lower (First Nations Health Authority n.d., 5).

Both CHIC and the health industry have started on a rather uncharted path of decolonization. Significant work has happened in the past two years with FNHA and Northern Health working together on primary care, mental health, and ER services. Although health care in general shares many founding principles, the Gitxsan health principles are firmly based in our traditional hereditary system. We already have in place incredible care and support systems within our families and communities. These systems are extremely practical, proven, inclusive, and trusted. CHIC views this planning as a way forward that would allow us to be part of the reconciliation conversation moving forward. CHIC's participation as independent community representation is seen as a counter to overlapping maps and jurisdictional gaps of the health care industry.

CHIC can offer partners practical solutions that reflect communities, research, data, demographics, and budgets, and has processes in place that create pathways to friendships, relationships, and a revolution in health care. Partners have to be prepared to work with each other and celebrate their relationships by working in a healthy range of reliance.

We will be allying with other provinces and Nations to help us gain insights, not just from their own personal and professional experiences but also as guests who have been asked to witness our transformation.

On Partnering and the Importance of Real Collaboration

My collaborator, Dr. Leslie Main Johnson, has been working in our communities since the early '80s. In the relationships that she has built over the years, including working with my grandfather, Ray Morgan, who was K'suu (a hereditary Gisga'ast Chief), she has shown to have commitment and responsibility to our communities and she has (as she should) intimate knowledge of the relationships within our hereditary systems and social infrastructure. She has learned what is important; it is not research projects and deliverables so much as research relationships, at least in working with and for our communities. We work together to define and move toward goals that are set in conversation, supporting each other, as we each bring our skills, interests, and histories to this conversation.

It is useful to us in our work to have a demonstrated connection with academic universities and researchers. It is useful to Leslie in her work, and even essential, to have community collaborators (e.g., a board or committee representing all Clans) to help maintain connection to places remote from where she now lives, to act as liaison, to help bring problems and opportunities to attention, and to keep Leslie's work grounded in the community and ethically aware. As part of a decolonization process, academic researchers cannot set research goals or targets independent of local priorities and in the absence of guidance. They must work in a spirit of sharing so that their work will have application and be useful in the community, as well as for academic purposes.

Research relationships are for the long haul. There are responsibilities to those who shared and share, past and present, to give back, to preserve, to help support usefulness. There are responsibilities to the future, as well as the present. Nations and communities are repatriating our knowledge (not just artifacts) and research, to reflect our ownership over knowledge. Using Traditional Gitxsan Public Health as a foundation for research will create a stronger basis for correct decolonized data and a way forward for implementing results within the Laxyip (territories), Galts'ep (communities), and Wilp Siipxw (Wrinch Memorial Hospital).

Communities and Nations need to be in control of the narrative moving forward. Gitxsan narrative post-contact is a very different experience than the people who came from away have documented.

The people who came from far away, left their families and became individuals, travellers forever shifting, for work, finding new homes and new families, on our Laxyip. Land and resources taken from the Gitxsan and freely distributed to the newcomers. Some non-Indigenous behaviour went beyond the forced immigrations of industrialization, wars and famines that forced them to immigrate here. Immigrants—people who came alone without grandparents. People who the Gitxsan took care of upon their arrival.

Translating our experiences, as Ermine (2007, 201) points out, can sometimes seem overwhelming, especially insofar as it "involve[s] and encompass[es] issues like language, distinct histories, knowledge traditions, values, interests, and social, economic and political realities and how these impact and influence an agreement to interact." We are those for whom this type of matriarchal community public health care knowledge was left generations ago, when people from away came to live with us. It is impossible for the "health industry" to replicate our matriarchal public health system that is our Nation's inheritance without us. The templates to healthy communities lie within each Nation and the Matriarchs.

The Gitxsan Treaty Office wrote in 1998:

> The Gitxsan *wilp* kinship system defines the roles, responsibilities and relationships wilp members have to one another...[We] seek to recognize, support and strengthen the wilp kinship network: *wilp, pdeek', wilksiwitxw, wilna'daahl, andim hanak, aye'e* and *ni'dils*.[15] (12)

Gitxsan knowledge, relationships, responsibilities, and roles become the point of reference for teaching and learning.

Matriarchal Inheritance (Clan, House, and Family)
Each Wilp (House group) and Pdeek (crest) has a very sophisticated Ayook (Hereditary Laws) that guides relationships, behaviours, and participation within the Wilp. Within Gitxsan traditional and ethical values, the extended family or Clan structure was once a very strong internal mechanism to overcome adversity, but the post-contact experience has caused the breakdown of the traditional systems to create dysfunction at the individual, family, and community level.

In order to preserve and protect their Daxget (power of the people), the hereditary system is solely responsible for the affairs and the well-being of the total Wilp membership. A complex interaction of obligations, sanctions, and mutual respect serves to maintain our society in relative harmony. There is equal access to resources, the house system, and consensual decision making. In 2006, the Gitwangak Simgiget[16] did a survey of the Wilp members and found that those who had a more traditional upbringing, participating in feasts, language, traditional foods, and the traditional supports in-place, thereby better knowing who they are and where they come from, tended to be more successful in education and careers.

The Gitxsan hereditary system provides us with a foundational template in place that the health care systems, including the health centres, can be integrated into. Supporting the Matriarchs is thus supporting the entire family, house, and Clan. Some terms are explained as follows:

- **Wilp**: Each Wilp has inherited assets handed down from generation to generation forever. *Wilnadehl*, laxyip, *adaawx, ayook, limx oo'ii*, and *waaim taa* are all part of the *gwalx yeens*[17] held by the Wilp.
- **Wilnadehl and Wilksiwitxw**:[18] Your own Clan relatives and your Father Clan, your support system from birth to death. Father Clan members make your cradle when you are born, and, when you die, they baptize all your names, take care of grave digging and washing the body, and are a lifelong important support system.

- **Galts'ep (community public health)**: Galts'ep means community. Community Public Health means supporting the individual, family, Clan, and House (Wilp) within the community.
- **Laxyip (territorial public health)**: The territories and who we are as a Nation provide a path forward.

The relationship to land, Laxyip, is fundamental. Culture camps on the Laxyip being used as trauma centres with mental health counsellors available on-site, with the supports of nature, art, and cultural overlays, providing ongoing resources that the communities can actually access and support, is an effective pathway to health. This conclusion is supported by important work undertaken by Chandler and Lalonde (2008):

> Taken altogether, this extended program of research strongly supports two major conclusions. First, generic claims about youth suicide rates for the whole of any Aboriginal world are, at best actuarial fictions that obscure critical community-by-community differences in the frequency of such deaths. Second, individual and cultural continuity are strongly linked, such that First Nations communities that succeed in taking steps to preserve their heritage culture, and that work to control their own destinies, are dramatically more successful in insulating their youth against the risks of suicide. (7)

Conclusions

The Gitxsan Traditional Health Plan utilizes work in the communities and on the territories. I have described above how the Tam Gisst Culture Camp was effective in reaching many health goals, and culture camps are an important strategy for community healing. Key goals in effectively creating culture camp/trauma centres include the following:

1. Re-establishing our Matriarchs as leaders and supporting intergenerational relationships that historically have supported all areas of individual and community health and wellness—physical, emotional, psychological, and spiritual.

2. Increasing connectivity of youth and Elders in the community, with a greater awareness among youth of health and wellness-related issues and their ability to contribute to a healthier community.

3. Involving individuals, families, and community members through active participation in traditional activities, connecting to local resources and assets, existing strengths, assisting to achieve and support their wellness objectives.

4. Reduction in the prevalence of addictions (alcohol and drugs) issues, with a specific focus on individuals, family, and community, and reduction in behaviours and social/familial issues that are correlated with drug and alcohol misuse/addiction. Reduction in the number of undiagnosed, unsupported, and isolated people who have mental health issues. Providing safe spaces for firefighters, first responders, paramedics, and others to recover from trauma and PTSD.

In this approach, trained mental health and Traditional Healers staff the camps and provide programming, enabling the clients to get out on land to heal and come together.

In addition, establishing effective regional access to culturally safe emergency and hospital care is key to Gitxsan public health planning. Wilp Siipxw (Wrinch Memorial Hospital) must be integrated with and work within our Gitxsan Traditional Public Health system to the benefit of all.

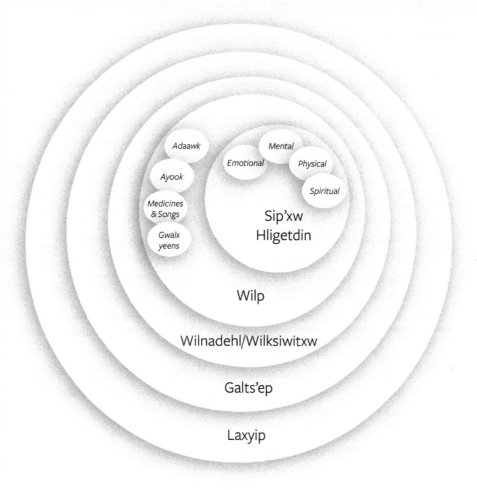

FIGURE 6.8 *Traditional Gitksen system linking people with social and ecological structures.*

1. Many people have contributed to this work, including Ray Morgan, Beverley Anderson, Naomi Himech, Ken Mowatt, Art Mathews Jr., Amanda Zettergreen, Joanne Daniels, Sylvia Johnson, Frances Jackson, Frank Shannon, Geoge Muldoe, Ann Howard, and Leslie Main Johnson. I am thankful for their help and have transcribed and documented the wisdom they have shared.

    Thank you to those who have expressed these ideas in the past, as Gilawo'o, Peter Turley, says, "We have done this in the past; the papers are in boxes at the Gitwangax Education Society and a few people have them stored in their houses." These ideas have a long history of being planned and put forth, but not consistently, practically supported, and implemented throughout the Galts'ep (community) and Laxyip (territories) by all.

2. Liliget is the feast hall, where feasts (Potlatches) are held and all-important traditional business was and still is transacted.

3. Unist'ot'en is the Wet'suwet'en resistance encampment on the territories on the Wedzin kwah (Morice River), which blockades the LNG (liquified natural gas) pipeline route through the mountains to Kemano on the British Columbia coast (see http://unistoten. camp/). It has subsequently become prominent in the struggle to maintain territorial sovereignty and resist unilateral and destructive resource development on their *yintah* (land or territories).

4. All unattributed epigraphs within this chapter are the author's own words.

5. The First Nations Health Authority is directly funded by the federal government through the First Nations Health Council.

6. The spelling "Gitxsan" has become accepted for the Nation as a whole. "Gitksen" is the spelling in the Geets dialect. Gitwangak is a Geets village.

7. For example, see the 2018 news release regarding a memorandum of understanding regarding establishing a satellite dialysis unit at this hospital at https://allnationshealing-hospital.ca/.

8. The term *wilaa luu t'aa goot* (knowing from the heart) was provided by Sim'oogit T'enimgyet, Dr. Art Matthews, at the health plan planning workshop in Gitwangak , February 2013, to indicate a healthy and whole mental state.

9. Anthropologists distinguish *matrilineal* (inheritance, titles, and territories passing through the mother's line) from *matriarchal societies* (government by female persons of authority). Here I recognize inheritance through the mother's line, women of authority, and the guiding role of women, and the fact that Sigidim Hannak and Sigidim Haanak are now most often translated as Matriarch or Matriarchs. Formerly, Sigidimnak was often rendered as "Chieftaness" in English. I am not concerned with formal classifications of political

structures in the present context but recognize the power and status of women in traditional Gitxsan and other northwestern Indigenous societies.

10. Wrinch Memorial Hospital is the hospital in Hazelton, BC. It was established by the medical missionary Horace Wrinch in the early twentieth century, and remained a private, church-run medical facility until 2016. See Johnson, Chapter 3 in *Wisdom Engaged: Traditional Knowledge for Northern Community Well-Being* (2019) for a discussion of the mission period, Dr. Wrinch, and the efforts to suppress Gitxsan and Wet'suwet'en healing traditions in the early twentieth century. A biography of Dr. Wrinch, *Service on the Skeena: Horace Wrinch, Frontier Physician*, by Geoff Mynett, was published in 2019.

11. The *Sixties Scoop* is the term given to the removal of large numbers of First Nations children from their families who were put in foster care, generally with non-First Nations families, alienating them from their families, cultures, and identities, and often exposing them to unstable and substandard care conditions.

12. See the *Globe and Mail* article detailing the inequities of treatment of First Nations children and the judgment of the Human Rights Tribunal (Grant 2016).

13. See Grant (2016) and *The Interior News* (2016) describing the out-of-court resolution of the class action suit brought before the BC Human Rights Tribunal for discrimination in quality of health care for First Nations patients at Wrinch Memorial Hospital.

14. Discussion of aspects of traditional Gitxsan modes of illness treatment can be found in Johnson (1997, 2006, 2019).

15. This list of basic terms of social relationship includes *wilp* (house), *pdeek* (crest), *wilksiwitxw* (father's side), *wilnadehl* (mother's side), *antim hanak̲* (spouse's contribution), and *ay'e*, which is the payment of the grandchildren to the father Clan during their feasts that helps pay for use of their grandfather's territory, and *ni'dils*, which apparently refers to the mother's side. These spellings are in the Gigeenix or upriver dialect, and some differ from the Geets spellings.

16. The plural of Sim'oogit, Chief, in the Gitxsan language.

17. Each individual belongs to a Wilp through inheritance on the mother's side, which owns its laxyip. Adaawx is "true tradition," oral histories of the House; ayook means law; limx oo'ii is the inherited mourning song of a key ancestor of the House; gwalx yeens is the inheritance of the House, the real and intellectual properties of the house.

18. Wilnadehl (the Geets spelling) are the relatives on the mother's side; Wilksiwitxw are the relatives of the father's side, the Father Clan members who have many reciprocal responsibilities.

REFERENCES

Chandler, M.J., and C.E. Lalonde. 2008. "Cultural Continuity as a Protective Factor against Suicide in First Nations Youth." *Horizons* 10, no. 1: 68–72.

CHIC (Community Health Improvement Committee). n.d.b. Policy Brief, First Nations Hospital. Unpublished document in CHIC files.

CHIC (Community Health Improvement Committee). n.d.a. Research Proposal. Unpublished document in CHIC files.

Daly, R. 2005. *Our Box Was Full: An Ethnography for the Delgamuukw Plaintiffs*. Vancouver: UBC Press.

Dell, E.M., M. Firestone, J. Smylie, and S. Vaillancourt. 2016. "Cultural Safety and Providing Care to Aboriginal Patients in the Emergency Department." *Journal of Emergency Physicians* 18, no. 4: 301–5.

Elias, B., J. Mignone, M. Hall, S.P. Hong, L. Hart, and J. Sareen. 2012. "Trauma and Suicide Behaviour Histories among a Canadian Indigenous Population: An Empirical Exploration of the Potential Role of Canada's Residential School System." *Social Science and Medicine* 74: 1560–69.

Ermine, W. 2007. "The Ethical Space of Engagement." *Indigenous Law Journal* 6, no. 1: 193–203.

First Nations Health Authority. n.d. *First Nations Health Status & Health Services Utilization: Summary of Key Findings, 2008/09–2014/15*. First Nations Health Authority, Coast Salish Territory, West Vancouver, BC. https://www.fnha.ca/Documents/FNHA-First-Nations-Health-Status-and-Health-Services-Utilization.pdf.

Gitxsan Health Society. 1986. Appendix M: Traditional Medicine. Gitxsan Health Society, Health Plan submitted to Health Canada. On file, Gitxsan Health Society, and in the files of the author.

Gitxsan Treaty Office. 1998. *Taking Stock: Watershed Inventories, Analysis and Planning, a 5-Year Capacity-Building Plan 1999 to 2004*. Gixsan Treaty Office, Hazelton, BC. Unpublished report on file.

Grant, T. 2016. "Cindy Blackstock, Canada's 'Relentless Moral Voice' for First Nations Equality." *The Globe and Mail*, July 14, 2016. https://www.theglobeandmail.com/news/national/cindy-blackstock-canadas-relentless-moral-voice-for-first-nations-equality/article30915894/.

The Interior News. 2016. "Settlement Reached in Wrinch Lawsuit." *Interior News* (Smithers, BC), January 6, 2016, A-18.

Johnson, L.M. 2006. "Gitksan Medicinal Plants: Cultural Choice and Efficacy." *Journal of Ethnobiology and Ethnomedicine* 2, no. 29 (June 21). doi:10.1186/1 746-4269-2-29.

Johnson, L.M. 1997. "Health, Wholeness, and the Land: Gitksan Traditional Plant Use and Healing." PhD dissertation, University of Alberta, Edmonton.

Johnson, L.M. 2019. "Illness and Power in Times of Contact: Gitxsan and Witsuwit'en Narratives of Healing." In *Wisdom Engaged: Traditional Knowledge for Northern Community Well-Being*, edited by L.M. Johnson, 51–84. Edmonton: Polynya Press.

Johnson, L.M. 2010. *Trail of Story, Traveller's Path: Reflections on Ethnoecology and Landscape*. Edmonton: Athabasca University Press.

Kelm, M.-E. 1998. *Colonizing Bodies: Aboriginal Health and Healing in British Columbia, 1900–50*. Vancouver: UBC Press.

Kirmayer, L.J., C.L. Tait, and C. Simpson. 2009. "The Mental Health of Aboriginal Peoples in Canada: Transformations of Identity and Community Healing Traditions." In *The Mental Health of Aboriginal Peoples in Canada*, edited by L.J. Kirmayer and G.G. Valaskakis, 3–35. Vancouver: UBC Press.

Marsden, S. n.d. *An Historical and Cultural Overview of the Gitksan* (2 volumes). Unpublished report to the Gitksan-Wet'suwe'ten Tribal Council, circa 1987.

Marsden, S. 2008. "Northwest Coast *Adawx* Study." In *First Nations Cultural Heritage and Law, Case Studies, Voices, and Perspectives*, edited by C. Bell and V. Napolean, 114–49. Vancouver: UBC Press.

Mynett, G. 2019. *Horace Wrinch, Frontier Physician*. Vancouver: Ronsdale Press.

Oster, R.T., A. Grier, R. Lightning, M.J. Mayan, and E.L. Toth. 2014. "Cultural Continuity, Traditional Indigenous Language, and Diabetes in Alberta First Nations: A Mixed Methods Study." *International Journal for Equity in Health* 13: 92. https://doi.org/10.1186/s12939-014-0092-4.

Saskatchewan Health Authority. 2018. "All Nations' Healing Hospital—Saskatchewan Health Authority Sign Memorandum of Understanding." News Release, Thursday, October 18. https://www.saskhealthauthority.ca/news/releases/Pages/2018/Oct/ANHH-SHA-sign-Memorandum-of-Understanding.aspx.

Truth and Reconciliation Commission. 2015. *Honouring the Truth, Reconciling for the Future: Summary of the Final Report of the Truth and Reconciliation Commission of Canada*. https://ehprnh2mwo3.exactdn.com/wp-content/uploads/2021/01/Executive_Summary_English_Web.pdf.

United Nations. 2008. *United Nations Declaration on the Rights of Indigenous Peoples*. https://www.un.org/esa/socdev/unpfii/documents/DRIPS_en.pdf.

7   Holistic and Culturally Based Approaches to Health Promotion in Alaska Native Communities

GARY FERGUSON, MEDA DEWITT,
AND MARGARET DAVID

This chapter is based on a joint oral presentation by team members of the Wellness and Prevention Program of the Alaska Native Tribal Health Consortium at the Wisdom Engaged: Traditional Knowledge for Northern Community Well-Being conference, which took place in Edmonton, Alberta, in February 2015. The session was video-recorded, and the present text is an edited transcript of the presentation. Presently, Gary Ferguson is Director of Outreach and Engagement at Washington State University, Elson S. Floyd College of Medicine; Meda DeWitt is a Tlingit Traditional Healer, ethno-herbalist, multidisciplinary artist, and educator in private practice; and Margaret David is practising as a certified midwife with the Alaska Native Medical Center.

Gary Ferguson—Introduction

I am originally from Sand Point, a small fishing community of eight hundred people in the Shumagin Islands of the Aleutian Islands region of Alaska. I grew up commercial salmon and halibut fishing and spent a lot of time by the ocean. My Indigenous heritage as an Unangan/Aleut comes from my home region, and my grandparents, Emil and Marina Gundersen, are from Sanak Island. My father is not native to our region; he is from upstate New York near Canada.

I finished my doctoral training in naturopathic medicine in Portland, Oregon, in 2001, and I've been working in the Alaska Tribal Health System now for almost fourteen years [as of 2015]. I had the honour of serving my home region at Eastern Aleutian Tribes when I first became a naturopathic physician. I served nine village clinics situated within a nearly thousand-mile catchment area. The Aleutian region is very vast and isolated, known as the "birthplace of the winds." My work there has primarily been in diabetes prevention and general health promotion. I've also worked in leadership roles at the Alaska Native Tribal Health Consortium (ANTHC) in wellness and prevention and community health services, and I've had a clinical practice at Avanté Medical Center in Anchorage and continue to consult for tribal health organizations on integrative medicine and naturopathic medicine for the First Peoples of Alaska.

The Alaska Native Tribal Health Consortium serves all 229 federally recognized Tribes in the State of Alaska and collaborates with those Tribes through partnerships to promote healthy communities. There are also many small tribal health consortia throughout our state; for example, the Southeast Alaska Regional Health Consortium, Chugachmiut, and the Aleutian Pribilof Islands Association all serve our regions. The Alaska Native Tribal Health Consortium serves the entire state for tertiary care, but if you need specialty services—cardiology or oncology, or different kinds of specialty care—you come to our main hospital at the Alaska Native Medical Center in Anchorage.

Meda DeWitt—Introduction

My Lingit names are Tśa Tsée Náakw and Khaat kła.at. My adopted Iñupiaq name is Tigigalook, and my adopted Northern Cree name given to me by Elder Harry Watchmaker is Boss Eagle Spirit Woman, or "Boss" for a teasing nickname. My Clan is Naanyaa.aayí, and I am a child of the Kaach.aadi. My family comes from Shtuxéen kwaan (now referred to as Wrangell, Alaska). My family lineage also comes from Oregon, Washington, and the BC/Yukon territories. Currently, I live on Dena'ina lands in south central Alaska. I honour my Aan ax shawdat, Elder Della Cheney, who is Kaach.adi from Kake, who is my father's Clan sister, making us allied Clans.[1] Our great-great-great-grandmothers were sisters. I'd also like to give thanks to the community hosting us on the traditional lands of the Indigenous Peoples who are still here and who have been so gracious to allow us to be here. *Gunalchéesh.*[2]

I work with the ANTHC, Community Health Services, Wellness Division, Health Promotion, Disease Prevention (HPDP), as a program associate. I work under Margaret David, HPDP program manager, and then Dr. Gary Ferguson, Wellness Division supervisor.

I am the co-chair, along with Margaret, organizer, and host of the Alaskan Plants as Food and Medicine symposium, organizing and facilitating the training of individual and community capacity-building trainings on Alaskan Plants as Food and Medicine, with over five hundred people reached. I also have been part of the Alaska Native Digital Storytelling trainings as a trainer and facilitator, organized and delivered the Women's Rites of Passage pilot project, and provided content editing and co-authored the *Doorway to a Sacred Place* guide and community outreach and education. I work as a Traditional Healer, representing and helping to translate Alaska Native traditional values, ideals, customs, and wisdom into contemporary social, educational, political, business, media, and economic venues.

Margaret David—Introduction

Margaret's introduction was not recorded due to technical difficulties. Margaret David was born and raised in rural Alaska. She grew up spending summers at her grandparents' fish camp on the Yukon River and is rooted by her Koyukon Athabascan culture. At the time this chapter was written, Margaret David was ANTHC's program manager, Health Promotion, Disease Prevention, and led digital storytelling workshops that taught Alaskans how to effectively tell their stories using modern tools. She also monitored the Alaska Native Center for Digital Storytelling website, which houses more than one hundred videos made by community members on topics as broad and personal as suicide, subsistence, spirituality, and culture. "Storytelling is a tradition in Indigenous and Native cultures and we help blend that with modern technology...What's really exciting about digital storytelling is that it's real people telling their stories firsthand, using their voice and experiences.

Viewers really relate to those personal experiences" (ANTHC 2012b, 4). Her section on digital storytelling follows Gary Ferguson's discussion of ANTHC and holistic health promotion.

Gary Ferguson—ANTHC and Holistic Health Promotion

At the Alaska Native Tribal Health Consortium, we have a vision of Alaska Native People being the healthiest people in the world. This vision is about wellness, not just the absence of disease. However, in Alaska, there is a dependency on outside food, and so a lot of our efforts are to address food insecurity. We define *food insecurity* as the inability to access sufficient, safe, and nutritious foods in socially acceptable ways. Food insecurity is higher in low-income populations, but in Alaska it is not limited to low-income people. There is an across-the-board dependency on outside sources of food. Statistics show that 104,510 Alaskans (14.6 per cent) are food insecure, including 36,670 Alaskan children (Food Bank of Alaska n.d.).[3] Children are disproportionally affected, and this is something that isn't going away when we look more closely at the problem.

To investigate the extent of food hardship, the Food Bank of Alaska carried out a survey of Alaskans in 2011 (Sullivan 2015). We asked one question in our survey: "Have there been times in the last twelve months where you did not have enough money to buy food that you or your family needed?" Of those surveyed, 18.2 per cent of Alaskans answered yes, and in 2015 19.2 per cent answered yes. This means that almost 20 per cent of Alaskans across the board experience food hardship. The problem is not limited to our Native population, but our interest here is in traditional foods.

The ANTHC worked with the Yukon–Kuskokwim Delta region of Alaska in a research project called Helping Ourselves to Health (ANTHC 2012a; Sharma et al. 2015; Kolahdooz et al. 2014). We give thanks to our Yup'ik leadership and communities for encouraging participants to be involved in the study. The study found that traditional foods are really nutrient-dense. However, in many of our communities, people are not getting the nutrition they need because of a diet shift with the adoption of processed and purchased foods.

An important concept in community nutrition and health is nutrition insecurity. *Nutrition insecurity* is having adequate (or even excess) caloric intake, yet still not meeting daily nutritional needs (ANTHC 2012a). This occurs when nutrient-dense traditional foods are replaced by high-calorie, but nutrient-poor, store foods. Traditional Alaska Native diets are very high in healthy fats, high in healthy proteins, and low in carbohydrates. We see the increase in preventable chronic diseases that are rising in our population as being directly connected to nutrition and changes in diet.

Colonization impacted and continues to impact our communities in many different ways. The time of contact varies across Alaska. In the Aleutians, the time of contact was around 1740, while in the interior it was some one hundred years later, with many villages only being first introduced to outside influences in the 1840s. This means that people from different areas of Alaska are in different places or stages in their adaptation to colonization. Colonization had many effects on people's health across Alaska. For example, there are challenges in accessing adequate nutritious food in communities where there may be 75–85 per cent unemployment. Obtaining country foods[4] is also costly, and people may lack the resources needed to go out on the land or sea to obtain their own food. One possible avenue to financial support is to use food stamps to underwrite resources needed to harvest food from the land, but many people are unaware that this is an option.

Access to clean, healthy water is another issue, and at ANTHC we also support a number of clean water and sanitation projects. There are some significant challenges like the impact of mining on local water quality. This is a substantial problem in southeast Alaska, where pollution from mines in British Columbia causes downstream problems with water quality. This is also spiritually problematic, as water is sacred, so resource development poses a real challenge. Lack of available, high-quality drinking water has also caused many problems. In the Aleutians near my home, there is a place called False Pass where the water is termed, "Sweetwater." Boats empty their freshwater tanks to take on water there. There is a need for infrastructure to support and transport high-quality drinking water. It is problematic that pop is cheaper than water and more accessible, as this makes addressing the high intake of soda an issue, especially in our villages. Some communities have substantial problems with dependency on soda pop, which undermines nutrition and increases risk of diabetes. In Barrow [Utqiaġvik] on the North Slope, which has a population of only four thousand people, they spend $1.5 million USD on pop every year.

Dr. Weston Price (1939) collected images of Alaska Native People in the 1930s. He documented how healthy everyone was.[5] His photographs show excellent dental health, as well as high infant and maternal health. There is a rich history of strong maternal/child health in our rural Alaskan communities that had vibrant cultures and foodways. His comments and images describe a very healthy people. There were no dental caries until store food was introduced. With the loss of traditional foods in the diet, there were not only dental caries but also changes in facial structure and dental arches—as a consequence of shifting to nutrient-poor, store-bought foods in place of traditional diets. The introduction of alcohol was also problematic, affecting nutritional health, as well as introducing new social problems. Alcohol not only robs the body of B vitamins but, as we know, drinking in early pregnancy can also cause fetal alcohol spectrum disorders.

Dietary changes also cause epigenetic changes. With diet change, there has been a 136 per cent increase in diabetes among Alaska Native People between 1990 and 2010 (Alaska Native Epidemiology Center 2014; see also Ferguson 2017; Ferguson and Bergeron 2013). Popular foods like fry bread and Spam contribute high amounts of salt and unhealthy fat, and, for fry bread, refined carbohydrates. These foods increase the risk of diabetes, unlike traditional foods such as seal or moose meat. Speaking of processed foods, Alaskans consume the second-highest amount of Spam per capita in the USA (Hawaii is the highest) (Brereton 2019). Processed meats are bad for our health, as they have excess salt, unhealthy fats, and preservatives such as nitrites. Unprocessed meat and fish, on the other hand, or meat and fish prepared without additives by home canning or freezing, are nutritionally superior and support health and well-being.

These health and dietary problems I have been discussing are all aspects of colonization, which have impacted and continue to impact our communities in a variety of ways. The effort to re-Indigenize our diet is a priority for promoting individual and community health in Alaska (Gilbert, Bergeron, and Ferguson 2017; Ferguson 2017; Ferguson and Bergeron 2013). Programs like the Store Outside Your Door, sponsored by ANTHC and our tribal partners, aim to increase knowledge of traditional foods from the land, how to harvest and prepare them, and how to introduce them to children and infants to help decolonize taste and promote healthy new generations.

Flour is refined carbohydrate, a type of food absent from traditional diets. Bannock, fried bread, is thought of as a traditional food but is not really a traditional food. It is a food of the post-contact period. Greens, fruits, and berries, on the other hand, are all traditional foods. Fireweed greens are nutritious and locally available. Foods like whale meat are high in healthy fats, proteins, and iron—nutrients not found in poor-quality store foods. Fish are high in healthy omega-3 fats that protect against cardiovascular disease and other chronic diseases associated with the standard American diet. High-quality foods from the land are health promoting and can aid in recovery from diseases like cancer;[6] however, we need to ensure our traditional foods are safe and free from contaminants that would undermine our health.

There are also some genetic differences that impair tolerance of Western-style diets in our communities. Congenital sucrase-isomaltase deficiency (CSID), for example, is prevalent in some Alaska Native populations, including Yup'ik and Iñupiat, among others.[7] People with this condition cannot tolerate grains or processed sugars. Milk can also be problematic in the Alaska Native population; many people are lactose intolerant or have outright allergies to milk products. We need to introduce traditional foods to babies and children so they develop a taste for healthy foods, and so they avoid the debilitating effects of foods they cannot tolerate, which interferes with their healthy development.

One of the programs that the Alaska Native Tribal Health Consortium has initiated to help address these issues is the Store Outside Your Door, which promotes the knowledge and use of healthy and traditionally valued Alaska Native foods. The aim of Store Outside Your Door is to assist communities in reinvigorating traditions that remind us how to hunt, fish, gather, and grow our own food. We also take an integrated perspective that views food as medicine, and Nature as medicine. We organize an annual event called Alaskan Plants as Food and Medicine, where people come together to share information on

Alaskan plants as food and medicine, and where we consider holistic and culturally relevant ways of health promotion. The program also sponsors a YouTube channel (ANTHCStoreOutside) to share video webisodes we produce that teach young families about traditional foods, demystifying their preparation for younger people, and incorporating these foods into modern recipes in a format similar to many shows on the Food Channel. For example, one webisode is about making Ky'woks [smoked sockeye salmon jerky strips] for teething infants in Metlakatla, Alaska.[8] The webisode demonstrates how to make the strips by processing salmon in traditional ways to feed families. It was produced by Desiree Jackson and me [Gary], working in tandem with the Southeast Alaska Regional Health Consortium and the Metlakatla Indian Community. We focused on the local food system and the local Tsimshian, Tlingit, and Haida Alaska Native People.

Store Outside Your Door also sponsors culture camps that teach not only about food but also feed resilience through cultural ways that aid in domestic violence prevention and substance abuse prevention. Studies show that when youth are connected to their culture and Elders, they are more resilient and less likely to engage in risky behaviours (The People Awakening Project 2004). In terms of population health, we have also produced the Ky'woks "Traditional Infant Feeding Guide"[9] I just described, and are working with our young people, getting the next generation set up for food preferences that sustain health. Our goal is to help young people get connected to our Store Outside Your Door program so they can learn more about their food traditions and local food system.

Protecting our waters, honouring our land, and making sure we have secure food and water for our future generations are traditional Alaska Native values. Because our health is so intimately connected to our environment, several ANTHC initiatives are focused on monitoring our changing environment, and all of our programs are targeted to support these traditional values.

Since a lot of our young people are on digital devices nowadays, we also recognize the importance of reaching our target audience—young Alaska Native families—through social media and technology and engaging with them on these online platforms. One young student in Galena [Alaska] created a digital short story about a Store Outside Your Door class that we were able to post on our YouTube channel, ANTHCDigitalStories.[10] It is interesting to note, however, that it is actually the older Alaskans who are engaging with our online programming the most right now. That makes us happy because it shows that Elders and "Elders in training" feel this programming is valuable and is a priority for us to share with future generations. They're the ones who are helping our next generations be connected to our work.

Meda and Margaret are the co-chairs of the Alaskan Plants as Food and Medicine symposium mentioned previously. One of the concerns the group has is how to safeguard and protect the information shared as a part of Store Outside Your Door. Dr. Rita Blumenstein, a Yup'ik Tribal Doctor and our mentor at the ANTHC Prevention Division, has told us it is time to share, but that we also must protect the knowledge of our people.[11] There is an economy around medicines, especially for our own people. ANTHC would like to see traditional medicines available in all medical centres accessible to our tribal members. There is a fear of traditional Ceremonies among people who had no exposure to such practices when they were growing up, and many trust allopathic doctors and Western medicine first.

We also work with the US Fish and Wildlife Service and the Alaska Department of Fish and Game to help ensure vibrant and viable animal and fish populations to enable sustainable access to traditional foods. Dialogue is needed, however, to keep our food system and access to it strong. We have gratitude for our non-Native allies from these departments, which is a part of our value system, who help to maintain the animals and plants we depend on. The premise is that we should share information, but in an ethical way. We need to teach people how to harvest, and how to be allies, to become a part of our family.

Margaret David—The Digital Storytelling Initiative

Another really important initiative in health promotion also uses digital technology. Our health promotion and community outreach programs focus on traditions and cultural knowledge, and one of the ways we reach out is through digital storytelling. As we serve the whole state, we focus a lot on supporting community health workers, so we're not necessarily doing the front line work but supporting those out in the community who are doing that work. A lot of these workshops that we've done are with different community health workers from all over the state.

A digital story is a short, one-to-three-minute video, usually. It's somebody telling their first-person experience, their first-person story. So, when they come to the workshop, we'll help them facilitate and put the pieces together and get through the workshop, but we don't tell the story for participants. Everybody makes their own digital story. It's really trying to get the community voices out there, so we can hear it from the people directly.

I've been with the health promotion program for almost five years now and I learned digital storytelling from the person who was there before me, and from Gary, and from some other people that got it started. I kind of took it on when I got started there almost five years ago. Since 2008, there have been over fifty workshops and over three hundred stories collected, so we're really rich in all these digital stories. We have a website where we house them online so people will have access to them. People have given permission for us to upload them there. We'll share that website with you, so people can view these stories and can be impacted by them, and also use them in their community health work as well.[12] I'm going to share two stories as examples.

This story that I'm starting with is by Grandma Madeline Williams. She's from the interior of Alaska as well [same region as Margaret], and she's one of our Elders and main culture-bearer and language teacher in our region. We're really honoured that she participated in this workshop when we went out to Hughes [Alaska] a few years ago. That workshop—I love all the workshops that I do, and that one was kind of one of my favourites just because of how organically it all came together. The person that brought me out there, he'd been talking to me for a couple of years about coming out, and so finally it came together that I was able to travel out there. I was prepping with him, saying, "Make sure to enlist ten people in the workshop, so it's worth all our time and investment in this, and this is what we need to do to help recruit," and he's like, "Yeah, yeah, ok," and then we get there off the plane and arrive at the Tribal Council building, and I'm all excited, saying "Who's coming?" and he picks up the VHF radio and he's like, "Digital storytelling at the Tribal Council. Come on down at 11 o'clock," and it's like, "Nobody knows? Nobody's coming? This is a three-day workshop to finish a story." And twenty people came down! This is a tiny village of less than 150 people, and so we had a small room full of people. It was half Elders and half younger people. Some of the youth workers came and nine people stayed through the whole thing and finished their stories. We had a couple of Elders that finished along with the youth workers and it just worked perfectly with the Elders—you know, natural storytellers; their stories flowed, and then they encouraged the youth in telling their stories. Then, when it came to the computer work, the youth were really excited about that part and had fun with the technology and helped the Elders. So it's a really awesome way, you know, digital storytelling—it brings people together. Storytelling traditions and digital technology, and Elders and youth, and it's really fun. Here is Madeline's story:

My name is Madeline Williams.

My grandparents are William Attla and Annie Attla. My parents are George and Eliza Attla. My Grandma and my Grandpa is from Hughes. My Mom and my Dad is from Hughes. They moved to Hughes here because of trapping and fishing. I am the youngest one out of the Attla family. I have two sisters and five brothers. For some reason, my brothers always look up to me.

When I grew up, work was just like playing time for me, like come for dogs, and getting water. We didn't have no running water in those days. Summertime, we'll get water from the river. Lots of times we get water from we melt snow.

In my days, when we become a teenager, we stay in a room for one month. They never let us talk to no one. That was our future, so we can be lucky in the past. We never ate no hot food, like cooked meals. We just ate dried meat and dried fish and water, and after one month is up, then they let us out of the room and we'd go out and chop off an old piece of dried fish to keep our luck for the future, and we'd go back to our own whatever we were doing before then.

I moved to Hughes in 1962. Elwyn Williams is my husband. We had eight childrens together. We adopted two. We raised one granddaughter. From then on I taught my children the way I was taught. My Mother taught me. I stayed in fish camp every summer. I also tanned moose skin what I learned from my Mother. Moose skin is not easy to tan. Now I am teaching my grandkids the same way I teach my kids. We teach our kids to catch their first goose, chicken, or fish and then they give it to an Elder for their luck. Also our grandsons catch their first moose. We later make a dinner for them, so they can have their luck for their future. I also teach our grandkids how to sew hats, gloves, mittens, medicine bags, coin purse, sun catchers, slippers, tops, and also how to cook fish and meat, and cook berries and make jelly. I also teach Athabascan language. I love winter culture. I work in the school nine months out of the year.

Life is not easy. In my lifetime, after being married for twenty-six years, I took my five children and I moved to Fairbanks because of alcohol problems in my family. After a few years, we worked out things and we were back together for our grandchildren. We lost two boys by suicide. It was not very easy. It was life as tragedy. I thought at one time I was going to lose my mind, but I worked it out by praying really hard and try to think of good things for my grandchildren and my children.

Now, we're back together, and life is good, things are working out. We take our grandchildren out every day. There's my story. Thank you.

This digital story was created in a workshop by Alaska Native Tribal Health Consortium, July 2012. Special thanks to Google pictures; my kids, my grandchildren, Bill, Janet, Thelma.

The cool thing about capturing this little movie is that we can now bring Madeline around with us, and students from other schools where she is not able to travel can still see her and be impacted by her. So that's one of the cool things about digital storytelling. We hear back in our evaluations after doing the workshops that going through that storytelling process is very healing for a lot of people that come through the workshops. Getting at that heart level of telling your personal stories directly, when people watch it, it reaches the intellectual and emotional aspects of your being. Sharing information about resiliency and the importance of culture. You know the lessons that we pull out of these stories, it reaches us at a deeper level that we connect with, and we also hear back in the evaluations from people watching the stories that it impacts them, and they become inspired to make healthy choices. So that's some of the reasons we love digital storytelling and keep getting requests and requests and requests to do more digital storytelling.

Suicide prevention is another area that a lot of people have worked really hard in, and there are different programs in our Community Health Services Division. We have a behavioural health program, and they have suicide prevention funds. By remembering the things that make us strong, and connecting back to our roots that make us strong, this is how we're trying to get at it as well.

We have suicide prevention programs that include care lines for people to call with trained professionals on hand to respond if somebody needs help, along with programs to teach communities how to look for signs and how to support people who may be at risk for suicide. We had one trainer last year who trained over one thousand people in these techniques, you know, she just kept going to communities. So our ANTHC Community Health Services Division is a big family where we have people focused on many holistic strategies for addressing health promotion and disease prevention.

We are building upon the digital storytelling work in partnership with the Alaska Tribal Health System. For example, the Maniilaq region in north-western Alaska worked with George Provost and others to create an online program called Project Life. George Provost is the Project Life manager at the Maniilaq Association. A bunch of students from the Maniilaq region school districts created digital stories. It was funded with money for suicide prevention, but it wasn't called "suicide prevention," it was called Project Life. Students created their digital stories, and then in small communities students would share their digital story and the community would surround them with positive energy about their story. Digital storytelling can be used in a bunch of different ways to help promote health without necessarily saying "suicide prevention." It was reinforced by encouraging young people that "You are important," and the community surrounds them saying, "Hey, you're valuable and your story is important," which I think a lot of young people don't hear enough.

Project Life is a really awesome project. It was all based on Iñupiat values on how to live well. It truly was suicide prevention, as they engaged communities in digital storytelling workshops all around their region. There is another group in the interior of Alaska that is doing a similar program with their youth, also with suicide prevention funds. They bought a classroom set of iPads that can be checked out and used when somebody is going to be doing a workshop at the school. You can get the classroom set of iPads and we did. We taught the students how to do digital storytelling on the iPads, which were really easy to travel with.

To make a digital story, it's a three-day workshop, and we spend the first day in story development. So listen to the participants' stories and get an idea for what they are going to be making. We help each person think about their story, and then we sit in a story circle where everybody gets a chance to share their story and get feedback from the group in a very supportive, positive, and safe space. We're trying to really get at what the heart of the message is that they're trying to get across—what their story is. The story that is wanting to be told the most at that moment. Then we go into learning how to put it together on the computer. Everybody is at a computer, and they are first working on their script. And then we help them record their voice and start matching up their images to it. We sometimes tie it together with some music in the background, and our final project comes out to a two-to-three-minute video.

The second video we will share is about expecting a baby, which the creator titled "An Everyday Practice of Acceptance and Forgiveness":

I was so excited! I am having a baby. I remember begging in prayer to God as a child, "Please give me a baby of my very own to hold," and now I was expecting the birth of my very own child.

Well, we tried to make it work one last time, but our relationship had always been undeniably toxic, and some words, once said, can never be taken back, and even with help, it just wouldn't work. I was so afraid. A baby boy, I thought, the spitting image of his father? Now that my partner was gone, how could I accept this heartbreaking disaster? Why does it have to be this way? I never wanted it to be this way! I'm so disappointed and so sad. I'm so ashamed.

My dreams are shattered. I am so alone. Will I ever make a fair life for this baby by myself? What kind of life will this baby even have without a father or a real family?

I am his mother and I know the truth. I am a warm and loving person. I have a kind and generous heart. I have so much love to give. I make healthy choices and I love this baby. My baby will be smart and will be safe with me. I will do my best. I will take birthing and pregnancy classes to learn as much as I can about my choices and my body. I will not be ashamed to go to church again. I will ask for help and I will not be stressed about the future, but trust and breathe and practise acceptance every day. I am so grateful for this baby with this healthy, changing body. I am beautiful and desirable. My baby needs me. Hold on. Welcome the care and love and help from those who are here around us.

Welcome baby. Hug him close and feed him and pray. Learn to ask, "Will you pray for us?" and, "Will you pray with us, please?" Understand and have compassion for this child's complete heritage. Honour the roots that God gave to him, just as they are. Protect this boy. Protect ourselves. Protect our hearts. I am not afraid. I have faith and I am not alone. I am so excited for what our future holds.

I am grateful to God for you...Margaret, Melanie, Meda, ANTHC, Grace Cromarty, Linda Cromarty and Warren Cromarty, Charles Cromarty, Lindsay Cromarty. This digital story was created in a workshop by Alaska Tribal Health Consortium, August 2013.

A lot of times when we travel out to the communities, there's not a specific topic for the stories. Usually, they're about culture, or tradition and wellness in general. This workshop that she came to was a healthy family beginnings digital story workshop. I started doing these a few years ago to try to gather stories of strength around becoming parents and learning about healthy parenting. Everyone that came to that workshop was interested in that topic and had a story around that topic that they wanted to share. Sometimes there might be a tobacco cessation grant, and the funders want to gather stories around tobacco prevention that they can use in their group, so we'll try to frame it around that as much as we can—while also still being flexible to allow whatever story needs to come out to come out.

Sometimes in that story circle process people come with a story in mind—and we actually see this a lot with professionals working in the tribal and community health administration offices. You know, they have a story in their head that they are really set on telling, and it's about their work, but then we get in that circle, and you don't know what's going to come up and something else comes up needing to be told first, and so then it will all change. That might seem kind of scary, because they prepared to put this other story together, and then it all changes when you get there. But we get through it, we get everybody through it, and everybody finishes 99 per cent of the time.

Sharing the stories is a healing process. People come with a story that is really hard for them to tell, and they believe they're not going to give permission to release their story and share it publicly, and that's fine, but what I find is that most of the time, by the end of the three-day process, when everybody has finished their stories, and we've had a premiere where we watch everybody's stories together, everybody wants the world to see their story. By that point, they're ready to put it out there and want everybody to see it and learn from it, so it's really fun and awesome to see that development.

The roots of this kind of project grow from the Berkley Center for Digital Storytelling,[13] and since then, digital storytelling has been Indigenized. We have to give credit to Brenda Manuelito, who brought digital storytelling to us in the first place at ANTHC through the University of Washington Native People for Cancer Control. She's now working with Tribes in the American Southwest region in digital storytelling training, so it's a rich legacy that she has created. The ANTHC digital storytelling program continues to bear fruit. The Southeast Alaska Regional Health Consortium has a very active digital storytelling effort, capturing stories, and so it's the gift that keeps giving.

At ANTHC, we have pursued a number of strategies to support and enhance health and wellness, addressing nutritional adequacy through the promotion and use of Alaska Native foods, both from plants and from animals. These foods are economically appropriate, as well as culturally valued, and deal effectively with the specific genetic makeup of Alaskan populations. We have enhanced access to clean water, and have supported Tribal Doctors and Traditional Healers who work with local traditions and practices. We have addressed mental and emotional health through the innovative use of digital storytelling, which enables our people to share stories of overcoming struggles, of resilience, and passing on traditions. We have also explored the potential of videos and social media to share important information on health promotion and contribute to the revival of culturally appropriate foods. ANTHC works together with our tribal partners to embrace the emerging field of integrative medicine, which brings together the best of allopathic medicine, along with Indigenous ways of healing—addressing illness in a holistic manner that draws on Traditional Knowledge, foods and medicines, effective integrative therapies, and the respectful use of allopathic medicine to enable Alaska Native People to achieve health and well-being.

NOTES

1. Tlingit society is matrilineal, and divided broadly into two moities. These, in turn, are divided into Clan groups, and then into house groups. There are strong relationships between Clans as allies. Allied Clans generally married to each other, creating alliances with your father's Clan group. Society is characterized by relationships of allies and equal-opposite reciprocity, and there are important responsibilities that must be undertaken by the father's side. The Kaach.adi of Kake are related to the Kaach.adi of Wrangell. Two sisters were ancestral grandmothers of these two Kaach.adi groups, who are closely allied to the Naanyaa.ayi of Wrangell.

2. *Gunalchéesh* means "thank you" in Lingit.

3. This is a statistical estimate based on annual (since 2009) studies conducted by Feeding America, which uses existing data on poverty, unemployment, and the Consumer Price Index to estimate how many people are hungry and in need of food assistance. The numbers given here are based on studies from 2014; new information is now available for 2021 at https://foodbankofalaska.org/hunger-in-alaska/facts-about-hunger/.

4. *Country foods* are foods from the land and sea, such as meat, fish, shellfish, berries, and plants. These foods were the basis of traditional Indigenous diets. They are more nutrient-dense and lower in fats and simple sugars than alternatives available from stores in the North. These foods must be hunted or gathered, or shared by those who obtain them.

5.   Price was a Canadian dental surgeon who travelled all over the world throughout the 1930s to photograph Indigenous Peoples' dentition. In his book, *Nutrition and Physical Degeneration*, can be found paired images of "ancient Eskimos," who ate traditional foods, and more recent Alaska Natives who were consuming diets high in carbohydrates, and who demonstrated specific issues with dental arch development and high rates of dental caries.

6.   ANTHC produced a book entitled *Traditional Food Guide for Alaska Native Cancer Survivors* (see DeCourtney 2008) to guide Alaska Native cancer patients in the use of traditional foods to support their health and recovery.

7.   According to the Alaska Native Medical Center (2016), an estimated 3 to 10 per cent of Alaska Native newborns have CSID, which is inherited as an autosomal recessive. Other northern Indigenous populations also have elevated occurrence of this disease—3 per cent for Canadian Inuit and 5 to 10 per cent for Greenland Inuit—while those of European descent have a much lower prevalence (0.2%).

8.   The webisode, "Metlakatla Ky'woks," is available at: https://www.youtube.com/ watch?v=PT9XbgJuNMs.

9.   See Store Outside Your Door: Metlakatla, Alaska, Ky'woks, https://www.youtube.com/ watch?v=3Q-EoEHjfHE.

10. To watch Kayla's digital story, please visit https://www.youtube.com/ watch?v=3pPdG8oWIvM.

11. Concerns about safeguarding Indigenous intellectual property are widespread, a topic Marc Fonda examines in Chapter 10. Many Indigenous groups fear exploitation of their knowledge for commercial purposes by outsiders, a concern with historical validity.

12. The digital stories can be found on the ANTHCDigitalStories YouTube channel: https:// www.youtube.com/user/ANTHCDigitalStories. For a similar use of digital storytelling in Alaska, see McCoy (2016).

13. In 2015, the Center for Digital Storytelling became StoryCenter, which is still located in Berkeley, CA. For more information, see https://www.storycenter.org/.

REFERENCES

Alaska Native Epidemiology Center. 2014. "Copper River/Prince William Sound Region: Diabetes Increase." http://anthctoday.org/epicenter/healthDataArchive/factsheets/ CopperRiverPWS_Diabetes_Increase_11_01_2014.pdf.

Alaska Native Medical Center. 2016. *Pocket Guide to Alaska Native Pediatric Diagnoses: Review of Diagnoses Rarely Seen in Other Populations*. Alaska Native Tribal Health Consortium. https://yk-health.org/images/b/b3/Pocket-Guide-to-Alaska-Native-Pediatric-Diagnoses_web.pdf.

Alaska Native Tribal Health Consortium (ANTHC). 2012a. *Helping Ourselves to Health: Addressing Factors That Contribute to Obesity among Alaska Natives.* USDA Research, Education, and Economics Information System. https://reeis.usda.gov/web/crisprojectpages/0209495-helping-ourselves-to-health-addressing-factors-that-contribute-to-obesity-among-alaska-natives.html.

Alaska Native Tribal Health Consortium (ANTHC). 2012b. "Lights...Camera...Health! ANTHC Uses Video to Engage, Inspire and Provide Better Health for Alaska Natives." *The Mukluk Telegraph*, April–June 2012. https://anthc.org › 2012_mukluk_april_june_lorez2.

Brereton, P. 2019. "People in Hawaii Consume 7 Million Cans of SPAM Each Year." *Ke Alaka'i*, April 25, 2019. https://kealakai.byuh.edu/people-in-hawaii-consume-7-million-cans-of-spam-each-year-reports-spam-website.

DeCourtney, C.A. 2008. *Traditional Food Guide for Alaska Native Cancer Survivors.* Anchorage: Alaska Native Tribal Health Consortium.

Ferguson, G. 2017. "Bright Spots in Addressing Nutrition Insecurity among America's Indigenous Population." In *Food Insecurity and Its Impact on Diabetes Management: Identifying Interventions That Make a Difference*, National Diabetes Education Program Webinar Series, 49–52. https://www.cdc.gov/diabetes/ndep/pdfs/Food_Insecurity_Slides.pdf.

Ferguson, G., and D. Bergeron. 2013. *Healthy Eating for People with Diabetes via the Store Outside Your Door.* Indian Health Service, Division of Diabetes Treatment and Prevention. https://www.ihs.gov/sites/diabetes/themes/responsive2017/display_objects/documents/training_seminars/SOYD_Transcript_508c.pdf.

Food Bank of Alaska. n.d. "Facts about Hunger." http://www.foodbankofalaska.org/hunger-in-alaska/facts.

Gilbert, T., D. Bergeron, and G. Ferguson. 2017. "Helping Ourselves to Health: Addressing Factors That Contribute to Obesity among Alaska Native People." In *Food Insecurity and Its Impact on Diabetes Management: Identifying Interventions That Make a Difference*, National Diabetes Education Program Webinar Series, 53–91. https://www.cdc.gov/diabetes/ndep/pdfs/Food_Insecurity_Slides.pdf.

Kolahdooz F., D. Simeon, G. Ferguson, and S. Sharma. 2014. "Development of a Quantitative Food Frequency Questionnaire for Use among the Yup'ik People of Western Alaska." *PLoS ONE* 9, no. 6: e100412. http://dx.plos.org/10.1371/journal.pone.0100412.

McCoy, K. 2016. "Exploring Cultural Identity through Digital Storytelling." *Green & Gold News*, July 20, 2016. https://www.uaa.alaska.edu/news/archive/2016/07/campus-community-exploring-cultural-identity-resurrection-digital-storytelling/?a.

The People Awakening Project. 2004. *The People Awakening Project: Discovering Alaska Native Pathways to Sobriety.* University of Alaska. https://alaska-alliance.org/wp-content/uploads/2020/10/People-Awakening-Project_original.pdf.

Price, W.A. 1939. *Nutrition and Physical Degeneration.* Redland, CA: P.B. Hoeber.

Sharma S., E. Mead, D. Simeon, G. Ferguson, and F. Kolahdooz. 2015. "Dietary Adequacy among Rural Yup'ik Women in Western Alaska." *Journal of the American College of Nutrition* 34, no. 1: 65–72.

Sullivan, M. 2015. "What We Know and How We Know It: Food Insecurity in Alaska." Food Bank of Alaska Presentation. https://slideplayer.com/slide/5982599/.

8 Southeast Tlingit Rites of Passage for Women's Puberty

A Participatory Action Approach

MEDA DEWITT,

TŚA TSÉE NÁAKW/KHAAT KŁA.AT

Meda DeWitt is a Tlingit Traditional Healer, ethno-herbalist, multidisci-plinary artist, and educator in private practice. This chapter is based on a senior project she submitted in completion of her BA in liberal studies at Alaska Pacific University (APU) in 2017, and was helpfully edited for inclusion in this book by Jennifer Andrulli, a Yup'ik Traditional Healer. Baasee' to Margaret Hoffman David for co-organizing the 2012 Women's Rites of Passage Pilot Project in southeast Alaska. Quyana to Dr. Rita Blumenstein for mentorship on Yup'ik traditional rites of passage. Quyaana to Victoria Hykes-Steere from Meda DeWitt for advising and mentoring her APU senior project.[1]

Introduction

In August of 2012, a group of women gathered in southeast Alaska to go through a rite of passage process together. This gathering was the culmination of a yearlong, and in some cases a lifelong, journey of conducting Elder interviews, research, planning, and preparation for the event. This event is an example of Indigenous participatory action research. The experience was deemed highly valuable by the participants and assisted in their personal growth processes. They also viewed the return of traditional Tlingit rites of passage Ceremonies as fundamental to the healing of their communities and culture. The purpose of this chapter is to create a foundational review of literature on southeast Tlingit women's rites of passage and to document the participatory action research event, the Women's Rites of Passage Pilot Project (SE WROP). This documentation serves as a necessary building block in the process of creating literary, cinematic, and community facilitation resources that focus on the purpose and implications for use of women's rites of passage.

Tlingit traditional rites of passage are based on Indigenous perspectives of how to create a healthy human, family, community, and environment. Rites of passage are used as an intensive knowledge, wisdom, and skills transference process, grounding the participants in their cultural identity and sense of self. They mark someone's readiness to transition into their next phase of life or mastery. There are many rites of passage periods during a person's life, generally associated with major biological, psychological, or social transitions. The Tlingit are masters of the initiation and cultivation of biological processes for augmenting life's natural rhythms and cycles, facilitating the necessary actions to ensure successful transition into new identities, responsibilities, and expectations.

During a public address, Nora Marks Dauenhauer, Tlingit poet and distinguished language scholar, once said, "They don't make them like they used to." Her statement referred to the Protocols, training, and learned disciplines that were a foundation of Tlingit culture, which are not present in Western culture. During developmental transitions or maturation events, the Tlingit had a structured set of activities and customs that would be performed, which are referred to collectively as rites of passage. One of the significant rites of passage in a Tlingit's life was the maturation process known as puberty. During puberty Ceremonies, youth would go through a set of activities that strengthened the physical, mental, emotional, spiritual, and relational aspects of their being. Rites of passage, while having similar purpose, have structural differences and offered varying degrees of intensity for individual participants. These variations were determined by the form and function of an individual's biology, their anticipated communal roles and contributions, social and political climates, and by their environment.

Rites of passage have been refined over thousands of years as a method for creating grounded, connected, present, sentient, healthy, contributing, sovereign human beings, and healthy, thriving communities. Preparation for rites of passage would be integrated throughout the participant's life via stories, activities, lessons, observations, and by supporting family, Clan, and community members going through the process. The process of preparation and support generated anticipation for the participant, cultivating a willingness in the participant to go through the process, an understanding of what was expected, and a sense of accomplishment once the rite of passage was completed.

Indigenous Protocols often observe the cycles, phases, and patterns of Earth and the universe. These observations are seated within particular places and share multigenerational, "deep spatial" knowledges, leading communities to understand that if Earth and the universe are to continue, then they must be renewed through Ceremony (Whyte, Brewer, and Johnson 2015). The current degradation and/or loss of rites of passage and other Ceremonies among the Tlingit and other Indigenous groups is directly linked to the recent changes in social and political climates that have occurred due to Western contact, colonization, and assimilation.

Review of Literature

The Tlingit are legendary for their oratory, particularly their rich tradition of storytelling, which is used to bestow cultural wisdom upon listeners. Storytelling provides context and brings a deeper understanding to any given subject that is generally lacking in the written accounts of non-Indigenous explorers and outside observers. This means that the literature available to impart adequate understanding of the knowledge transmitted to the individual going through a rite of passage is extremely limited. While there are a satisfactory number of written accounts about the physical activities and structures of women's puberty customs, none offer even a basic understanding of women's wisdom, traditions, power, or their deep cultural knowledge. In the 1991 reprint of G.R. Emmons's early twentieth-century study of the Tlingit people, for example, editor Frederica de Laguna adds notes identifying places where the male explorers' and anthropologists' accounts were "exaggerated and inaccurate in some details" (Emmons [1911] 1991, 266).

We can glean some information, however, by examining the writing of European and American authors. The following observation comes from German ethnographer Aurel Krause (1972):

> At the beginning of puberty, a girl is secluded as unclean and, like the woman about to be confined, is put in a little hut of branches. Erman describes these huts as six to eight feet high with a barred opening toward the sea and the street and otherwise closely covered with green conifer branches. (152)

Nancy Turner (1979) further explains that the conifer branches were western hemlock (*Tsuga heterophylla*) branches, and she records that pubescent girls lived in these hemlock bough huts "for four days after their first menstruation" (116). Krause (1972) continues:

> In several they were sitting with averted faces, but in one a young slender girl showed without shyness a face smeared and dirty with soot and charcoal. Formerly this seclusion is supposed to have lasted a whole year, Veniaminof reported that Tlingit in the vicinity of Sitka had already shortened it to half or a quarter of the time. Now they are satisfied with even a shorter period or the practice is entirely abandoned. During the whole period of seclusion, the girl was not allowed to leave her narrow and dark prison except at night and then only when fully covered. She had to wear a hat with a broad brim so that she would not look at the heavens and make them unclean with her glance. Only her mother and her slave or her nearest female relatives were allowed to visit her and bring her food. (152–53)

To further understand the physical activities of this rite of passage, one can look to the observations of German explorer Georg von Langsdorff (1814), as described by Krause (1972),[2] who indicates that during this period girls had to observe the greatest deprivation and were only allowed to sip water through the wing bone of a white-headed eagle. Krause (1972) specifies that the limited water intake would occur only at night:

> At the conclusion of the period, if the girl belongs to an important family, the relatives give a feast at which the girl, clothed in new apparel, is brought before the assembled guests whereupon the serving of food commences. The slave whom the girl clothes for this feast obtains their freedom and the old clothes are destroyed. During the menstrual period every woman is secluded for several days (Veniaminof says three) in a special hut and is regarded as unable to perform any household duties. (153)

These trends of limited access to understanding are most likely due to the explorers themselves being men and the custom of interviews occurring generally with other men of the Indigenous population, making women's knowledge unobtainable. Another challenge is that anthropologists in the nineteenth and early twentieth centuries generally chose to observe Indigenous populations with only limited interactions, believing objective observations would reduce their influence on the behaviours of those observed. The Tlingit people are complex, with a highly developed and stratified society, defined customs, and social Protocols, most of which are not understood through simple observation and superficial means of interaction.

Again, we can review many early explorers' accounts and immediately understand that only physical actions and perimeters were generally observed. For example, in the passage from Emmons ([1911] 1991) that follows, it is clear that understanding of the most important aspects of the puberty rite of passage process is lacking; the author even admits his own limited understanding and that in the original explorer's accounts by placing a "[?]" in the text.

Girls' Puberty

At the first signs of puberty, the girl was confined in a small outbuilding or in a partitioned space near the parents' sleeping place inside the house for a period of four months. This might be increased, according to her social position, to a year and even longer. As she was considered unclean, this confinement was intended to appease the spirits [?]. The whole procedure was discussed and arranged beforehand. The girl fasted for the first four days, drinking water only in the evening. She ate on the fifth day and then fasted for four more days. During this period, her fingers were bound; she was not allowed to wash, comb her hair or do any work; only her mother or her attendant could see her. After this fasting period was over, however, she was visited by her female relatives and playmates. Throughout her confinement, her food was restricted to dried fish and meat, oil, and berries and no fresh seafood was permitted. She drank water slowly through a bone tube, made of the leg bone of a swan or goose. Around her neck she wore a suspended stone charm with which she scratched her head or body; fingernails were never used. (264–65)

Emmons ([1911] 1991) continues describing confinement and mentions that instruction on how to be a woman occurs during the rite of passage, but he neglects to describe the nature or procedures of the instructions:

Throughout her confinement, she was encouraged to keep herself occupied with those industries common to women, and she was instructed in those procedures and manners of her future life that she had not already learned through observation. She never went out in the daylight, but at night, with her face almost covered by a hat or hood, she might be taken out by her mother or aunt. (If she looked at the sky, it would storm.)

At the conclusion of her confinement, if the family was of high caste, her father gave a feast, at which time she was bathed and dressed in new robes, and the confinement hat (puberty hood) was exchanged for one smaller, which was hung with a fringe of fur that partly concealed her face. She was seated in the place of honor opposite the doorway. Her lower lip was pinched until it was numb and then was pierced by her father's sister or a female member of his family (lineage) with a sharpened bear claw or bone awl, and a small bone plug was introduced to keep the hole open. In honor of this occasion and as a demonstration of the position and wealth of the family, a slave might be freed. (265)

Emmons also quotes von Langsdorff's (1814, 133) 1805 description of the confinement of girls when they reached puberty, but neither author provides details of what the girl learns or is "employed" with doing:

> It is not uncommon when a young girl is grown up to shut her up, even for a whole year, in a small house by herself, at a distance from her family and acquaintances, where she is kept constantly employed: the idea is, that by this means she acquires habit of industry and diligence, reserve and modesty, which will afford the better chance of her becoming a good wife, and lay a solid foundation for wedded happiness. It is certain that industry, reserve, modesty, and conjugal fidelity are the general characteristics of the female sex among these people and form a most valuable distinction between them and the women of the more northern parts of the coast. (cited in Emmons [1911] 1991, 266)

Finnish naturalist and ethnographer Henrik Johan Holmberg (1855) followed von Langsdorff's travels and also recorded observations of Tlingit rites of passage. De Laguna makes an editorial comment paraphrasing Holmberg's observations (1855, 39–41) in Emmons ([1911] 1991) below:

> At the first signs of puberty a girl was confined in a dark, cramped place because she was considered unclean. She must not look at the sky, to prevent which she had to wear a hat with a wide brim. Confinement was formerly (before 1850) for a year, but the Sitkans cut it to six or even three months. At the beginning of this period, her lip was bored for the labret. All Tlingit women had a limping, crippled gait, in comparison to the proud, upright carriage of the men, which Holmberg could not explain. (266)

De Laguna also provides an editorial direct quote in Emmons's book from Whit M. Grant, a district attorney who recorded observations about "old customs" being abandoned while living in Sitka in May 1888. De Laguna comments, though, that Grant's account is "exaggerated and inaccurate," but that it provides an indication of the fact that the ritual was still taking place in the late 1800s. Grant's direct quote is provided below:

They have a small house, about six by six feet and eight feet high, in which is a small door and one small air hole six by six inches in one side. In this they lock up and keep their maidens, when showing the first signs of womanhood, for six months, without fire, exercise, or association. All of the world they see is through that six by six-inch hole, and all they get to eat, and drink is through it. It makes no difference to them whether it is summer or winter. How the poor creatures survive the ordeal I can't understand. When let out, if alive, they are free to get married, and are often sold when in prison, to be delivered to their future husband when the term of probation is over. (Emmons [1911] 1991, 266)

The conclusion can be made that the observation of puberty seclusion by Western colonizers and their misunderstanding, misinterpretation, and subsequent condemnation of it played a primary role in the abandonment and criminalization of this Ceremony, as well as others like it. Frederica de Laguna infers that there was more to the process of puberty rites than what meets the eye. "In addition to stressing puberty as a time for learning the skills demanded of adulthood, the Tlingit would not seem to have considered the girl only as unclean or 'polluting'... but as filled with power, dangerous to others, to the environment, and to herself" (editorial comment in Emmons [1911] 1991, 266).

Further challenges that emerge in the existing literature stem from the fact that most publications have been written by non-Indigenous people, which produces a skewed or limited understanding of Indigenous rites of passage. Literature written by outsiders who have been accepted as supportive to the cultural group under observation reduces the level of misunderstanding and misrepresentation, but still does not impart the deeper understanding that occurs within knowledge transference and experience of living traditions. For example, anthropologist Jenny Reddish (2013), drawing on the work of Aldona Jonaitis (1988), professor of anthropology and author who specializes in Northwest Coast art, compares the female Tlingit labret piercing tradition to the male Amazonian labret tradition. Reddish tries to understand the purpose of lip piercing and stretching in the context of cultural expression, both in its physical and nonphysical manifestations. Reddish acknowledges that previous authors have provided valuable insights regarding the connection of lip plugs with ideas about speech, sociality, food, and marriage (2013, 58). However, she chose to focus on the pain and impracticality of piercings. She infers that the medium of the lip labret was socially structured pain as a process of effecting social and behavioural shifts in the person being pierced.

As Jonaitis (1988) notes, however, in the case of Tlingit girls, the lip was pinched until numb and then pierced, and with gradual stretching over time, the actual pain experienced in comparison to other forms of socially structured pain would be minimal. The pain-based social transformation theory also overlooks actual physical experience, especially in the context of pain threshold, which can be and is manipulated through a series of events throughout a girl's life, including proper long-term breastfeeding as an infant and other activities that harden the body. Even with the numbing of the tissue, a piercing elicits a physiological response of pain relief, with the release of euphoria created by endorphins. In addition to reductions of pain and an increase of euphoric sensations, endorphin release modulates appetite, releases sex hormones, enhances the immune system, and reduces the effects of stress (Stoppler n.d.).

Facilitated experiences of pain and suffering are used as a tool by many Indigenous groups in the process of rites of passage. Pain is used differently in men's and women's processes because it is understood that women will experience more pain throughout their lives simply as a function of their biology and social roles. Because men do not experience menses, give birth, or have the same level of biological duty or social responsibility in raising offspring, they undergo facilitated activities that produce pain as a function of creating empathy and a limited understanding of what women experience throughout their lives.

From a perspective of receiving piercings and other body modifications, it would be more relevant to say that the euphoria is more successful at creating psychological and visceral associations with the experience of transformation. However, the most significant is the visual marker that communicates to community members that the rite of passage has been completed. They reciprocally adjust their behaviour, expectations, and level of respect toward the young woman. This social recognition creates a significantly intense experience, which supports and affirms the acceptance of the transition into womanhood. With intimate knowledge of the Protocols and Ceremonies of the Tlingit people, it can be surmised that the Tlingit were aware of how the body's responses worked and capitalized on the natural physiological and psychological responses to pain to help strengthen relationality with the community, environment, and spirituality.

Before the arrival of European travellers, missionaries, and traders on the northern Pacific coast, labret use was a widespread cultural trait and had been practised for at least four thousand years (La Salle 2013/2014, 140), suggesting high cultural importance and deeply embedded significance. The ornaments themselves were made in a variety of shapes and from a number of different materials, including stone (soapstone/steatite), slate, bone, and wood. They were sometimes inlaid with shell or copper (La Salle 2013/2014).

Labret use was linked to coming of age and the prospect of marriage; as Jonaitis (1988, 191) notes, most eighteenth- and nineteenth-century European authors who encountered the Tlingit agree that a girl's lip was initially cut following her first menstruation, and that it signified her marriageability. The piercing formed part of a lengthy rite of passage from asexual childhood to sexual maturity. The girl was first isolated from her family and made to sit as still as possible in a dark hut for up to a year (196). At the start of her seclusion, a woman from the moiety of the young girl's future husband—preferably her father's sister in this matrilineal society—cut a slit into her lower lip and inserted a small pin. Then followed a period of fasting and abstention even from drinking water, finally the young woman was "reborn" from the hut, and her first real labret was inserted at a "sumptuous feast" (191).

Reddish (2013) invokes Arnold van Gennep's cross-cultural theory of rites of passage to understand labret use. Van Gennep described three phases or sub-rites of "separation," "transition," and "incorporation." Reddish states, "Among the historical Tlingit, the insertion of the labret into a girl's mouth also accompanied a social passage: the ornament signaled her marriageability and nobility, and ideally she would be married off to an opposite-moiety man soon after emerging from ritual seclusion (Jonaitis 1988: 194–6)" (Reddish 2013, 68). Many of the published accounts of the lip plate bring attention to the power of the woman's words, especially living in the opposite moiety's house, where careless words could cause indignation, bringing strife and conflict. These social Protocols are necessary, but they make me ponder the power of *seclusion*, not the labret itself, in the process of behavioural maturation. It appears, then, that one of the functions of seclusion and fasting is to bring about greater understanding of suffering derived from deprivation of food and comfort, allowing a true appreciation and deep-seated gratitude for the provisions and shelter that the girl's husband and in-laws would provide. The mindful oration required by the labret would then uphold this process of humility and gratitude, reducing the ease or mistake of lipping off. Considering that marriages, especially those among the nobility, would be arranged, these processes would safeguard against indignation and lament for the comforts of her parents' home.

The duration of seclusion was not simply based on social status alone. The concept of social status in America is identified by monetary worth, while traditional Tlingit concepts of nobility or higher social status are associated with the level of responsibility and duty to the community, the environment, and the spiritual balance of the universe. The weight of one's words or one's behaviours is more valuable, with extensive social currency and power being garnered through alliance cultivation and acts of intense generosity. High-caste Elder women in Tlingit society are tasked with keeping the cultural knowledge, history, genealogy, migration stories, identity, and spirituality intact. As age increased, so did their identity as keepers and advisors of Protocol, including rites of passage. Their role in the community is to keep the universe in balance and maintain the fabric of reality.

In Julie Cruikshank's book *Do Glaciers Listen* (2005), puberty rites are mentioned in traditional stories associated with the movement of glaciers that were recorded in written fashion. These stories are associated with movements of ice that occurred from the Last Glacial Maximum to the Little Ice Age.[3] There were significant changes in the environment and landscape at these times, changes so quick and grand that they would require substantial amounts of power to invoke. For this reason, it is not a surprise that the Tlingit would associate these environmental changes with Protocols of first menstruation or puberty seclusion being broken. The story in Cruikshank's book merges with those told more recently by two Elders from the

Chookaneidí Clan, Susie James (in 1972) and Amy Marvin (in 1984), recorded in Tlingit and translated by Nora Dauenhauer (Dauenhauer and Dauenhauer 1987, 244–91, and Notes 407–31):

> All three...bring us to the heart of questions regarding social consequences of moving glaciers, because they take as their central theme issues of social responsibility. In each version, a secluded young menstruant foolishly calls out to the glacier as though her words had no consequences, triggering an advance that destroys the village. The story's impact lies in the choices people are forced to make instantaneously as the glacier advances with alarming speed. In one version, the girl's grandmother insists that she will remain at the site so that her grandchild can leave and go on to bear children—crucial for the survival of the clan. In effect, she takes responsibility for her granddaughter's flippant words. In the other, the young woman insists on remaining behind, accepting full responsibility for her actions and being unwilling to face the shame of living with the consequences her actions have unleashed on others. Whatever the outcome, the image of the "woman in the glacier" remains the embodiment of the current Chookaneidí clan title to Glacier Bay, a claim clan members say is verified by the fact that they paid for this place with the blood of their ancestor, the woman in the glacier. (Cruikshank 2001, 385)

Julie Cruikshank also recorded the connection between ice and women's puberty when Elder Kitty Smith (of Athapaskan and Tlingit ancestry) shared her life story with Cruikshank while in the Yukon:

> HUMAN LIFE CYCLES are also about transformation. When Kitty Smith describes jarring transitions from childhood to early adulthood and marriage, she frequently draws on icefields imagery about a colorless winter world where whiteness—of landscape and animals—signifies abrupt social adjustments. Her story "The Stolen Woman" traces the journey of a young woman who is moving on from the safety of childhood to a new stage of life. She has passed puberty and is already married when she is kidnapped and spirited beyond the immense snowy horizon, "[where] daylight broke, the time the sky lifted

from salt water...the other side." Relying on a range of practical skills she has learned during her training at puberty, she manages to outwit her captors, assist her rescuers, and even engineer her own escape. The successful rescue party retreats from the "winter side" by reversing direction and returning to the horizon where they "wait for the sky to lift up" and return to the "summer side." (Cruikshank 2005, 81)

While the understanding and context of Cruikshank's analysis of the Kitty Smith narrative are less subversive than the accounts of the early European explorers, it is still limited by lack of personal understanding of cultural context. When the story is told, inference of understanding is garnered through more than rote words, the Lingit language is monotone with tonal inflections changing the meaning or context of the words used, as well as the use of hand gestures and body language, and through the transmission of picture-based thought forms. The simple translation of Lingit to English modulates down the level of meaning and depth of understanding possible in the process of storytelling. As a juxtaposition, the comments by Nora Dauenhauer and an excerpt from a paper written by Liz Cheney (now Elizabeth Medicine Crow) illustrate the depth and richness that comes from a cultural insider's articulation of women's rites. They turn the story or explanations into an almost poetic format that is much closer to the parable style in which Lingit is spoken.

As a footnote in her and her husband's book, Nora Dauenhauer describes what "Someone in this condition" means. Notice how she describes the meaning of what is going on, describing the experience, removing the stigmatization that happens through a Western lens:

This is one of the great miracles and mysteries of life, and in many traditional societies women were and are considered to have great power, especially at this time. The power can also be unconscious and dangerous, and many ritual taboos often apply. In traditional societies, the onset of menstruation is also one of the great rites of passage in a woman's life, and in the life of the community. (Dauenhauer and Dauenhauer 1987, 421)

This trend of articulating living cultural understanding is also demonstrated in a paper written by Liz Cheney on becoming a mother (while this is not the puberty seclusion Ceremony, it is a transition into a new identity with responsibility and expectations, and is significant to the Tlingit):

All through the pregnancy, the expecting mother was being continually told by her grandmothers, aunties, and mothers the role and importance of being a mother. Many of the women from around the village would come by to wish the unborn child a safe passage from the land of the ancestors. The expecting mother would spend her days listening and learning the rhythms of motherhood. She would sit quietly in places she felt drawn to and describe the beauty to her child. Whenever she worked on anything, she would take the time to describe how and why she was doing it. It was believed that if she did not speak quietly to her silent observer inside and share with it beautiful songs and stories, then the child would be born with empty ears, always trying to make noise, and it would have empty eyes, unable to see beauty. (Cheney 2007, n.p.)

The tone in the different styles is noteworthy, with one being objective observation of physical structures and customs versus the subjective, intimate story of a Tlingit woman taught by her aunties expressing the lineage of wisdom. The intergenerational transference of knowledge through story is not only substantially richer than the explorers' accounts, it is one of the foundational activities that occur during the woman's rites of passage process.

Indigenous storytelling is a powerful tool used in traditional cultures to talk about challenging situations. Storytelling is a part of traditional psychology and assists people through the process of self-identification and decision making (DeWitt 2015). Storytelling creates a cultural identity that solidifies world view and foundations of spirituality, and imparts understanding of the world and their purpose within the world. The understanding of how a person fits into social structures and what Protocols they must follow allows the person to fulfill that role to the best of their ability, and this identity is reinforced by their worth being reflected back to them, through gratitude and reciprocity from other members and nature.

The Importance of and Special Needs of Teens

The process of revitalizing and establishing a cultural identity and solidifying Tlingit youth as members of their culture is paramount to the survival of the culture. To achieve this, active members of the culture will have an opportunity to work together and recreate, adapt, and embody what it means to be Tlingit, and in this case, a Tlingit woman. Even the concept of Tlingit woman is synonymous with strength, intelligence, beauty, and vitality. However, the social and health disparities associated with being Alaska Native do not reflect these truths. To change the trajectory of the future generations, key developmental times are necessary to access and assist in the formation of identity. In American psychology, Eriksons' developmental stage of fidelity—identity versus role confusion that occurs in adolescence at 13–19 years of age—is the time when this occurs. This is in congruence with the Tlingit understanding that this stage deals with the fundamental existential questions: Who am I? and What can I be? As they make the transition from childhood to adulthood, adolescents ponder the roles they will play in the adult world (Erikson and Erikson 1997).

Currently, Indigenous people suffer from health and social disparities at disproportionately higher rates than non-Indigenous people (Lines and Jardine 2019). These disparities are symptoms of the process of assimilation and colonization, which is still in effect today. These mechanisms of trauma can be understood in three modes: historical, intergenerational, and persisting. Historical trauma is the total collective emotional and psychological wounding over the lifespan and across generations, stemming from massive group trauma. Either acute or chronic occurrences can cause historical trauma (Brave Heart et al. 2011). Generational or intergenerational trauma causes wounds in new generations, from the trauma past generations still carry. These wounds are passed down in cyclical fashion through displayed behaviours and attitudes. They are also handed down through epigenetics—cellular memory.[4] Persisting trauma, social, economic, institutional, judicial, or other extenuating factors perpetuate the effects of historical or generational trauma, creating environmental triggers and reinforcement of original traumatic impacts (DeWitt 2015).

Adverse childhood effects (ACEs) are common. An ACE is defined as one or more parent in the household who displays behaviour or a traumatic circumstance that was experienced as a child. The list of items on the ACEs questionnaire are as follows: substance abuse, parental separation/divorce, mental illness, battered mother, criminal behaviour, emotional neglect, physical neglect, emotional abuse, physical abuse, or sexual abuse. A maximum total score of 10 is possible, but a 0 would be ideal. The ACE scores are significant because they have the highest predictability to gauge experiences of addiction, social dysfunction, chronic illness, and more. For instance, an ACE score of 4 or more increases the risk 4–12 times for alcoholism, drug abuse, depression, and attempted suicide (Felitti et al. 1998; Dong et al. 2004).

Trauma is no stranger to our populations, especially our teens. When trauma happens, it affects the developmental stage in which it happens, stunting growth in that domain. The effects are generally unseen/hidden and manifest in relationships, stressful situations, or the inability to thrive in life. The limbic system stores memory and elicits responses to triggers of that memory. Depending on the age at which the traumatic memory was stored, the implicit and explicit memory or both will be triggered. When toddlers reach their teen years, the same behavioural stages and dysfunctional attributes reoccur. If the trauma occurred before the age of remembering, addressing negative behavioural manifestations can cause particular challenges. Parents, family, and community can prepare by reviewing and assessing what worked and what did not for that person in their toddler years.

Teens are in a rapid state of growth and change, in both the body and emotions. The teen brain is in chaos. To feel normal, they may engage in either negative or positive management systems. The negative management systems would be to create chaos to match their internal world, through self-medication/mutilation, or tuning out. Positive management systems involve directing energy into solving problems, or by challenging themselves with physical or mental tasks. Challenges require planning and organization and can help the brain to unwind and calm the storm if the teen has been taught how to conduct the process. Teens are in a stage of social development and understand themselves by understanding their peers; they tend to harmonize with the group or surroundings as a natural function. The journey of the body helps the journey of the mind and emotions, trials and learning create experience, maturity, and wisdom. The internal or external journeys were traditionally facilitated through rites of passage.

From an Indigenous cultural view, teens are supposed to be the way makers, expected to test their environment, meant to find new ways to do things. Elders and communities looked to that age group to inform and improve the way things are done. Teens look for hypocrisy with a razor-sharp critical eye, constantly looking for incongruence or the weak link in the chain. Once they believe something is worth idealizing, they will then overlook flaws and can even emulate them as part of the image. They do not want to be incongruent from their peer group, because then they are the anomaly and will be picked off. Testing identity of likes and differences leads to the emulation of and idealization of people. Images that are generally sought after to emulate are: strong; fast; hard; no fear; master of environment, body, and emotions; and have some sort of power or influence over their peer group. Rebuilding rites of passage will develop from the basics of teaching them how to be a "bad ass" through testing their own skills, using a litmus test worthy of their vitality, Mother Nature, and themselves.

Strengthening our young adults to be ready for rites of passage starts long before the beginning of adolescence. Even the simple fact that America has high rates of C-sections and low rates of breastfeeding weakens our population. Because breastfeeding and positive caregiver attachment builds stronger humans for life. Both actions positively reduce pain perception, teach trust, create attachment, enhance better-formed brains and gray matter, build resilience to stressors, and reduce chronic health issues. Healthy role models create and/or reinforce these same benefits.

The Western term "behavioural health" can be replaced with the Indigenous concept of *relational health*. We learn about ourselves by cycling through inward and outward relationships. We are social beings that use mirror neurons/axons, hormonal responses (oxytocin, endorphins, gonadotropins) to social stimuli, and rearing techniques (skin to skin, a mother's love is the best pain killer, breast milk, etc.) to create strong social networks and healthy people.

Rites of passage can assist in healing from trauma and the transition into adulthood by rebuilding an individual. Even through relationship building with plants, trust relationships can be created with Mother Earth. Touch is necessary, therapeutic touch with permission, and is done correctly when the female attendants do things such as brush the participants' hair, massage their hands or back, or even just sitting in proximity. Mentors—or honorary uncles and aunties to the kids—recreate positive social bonds.

Teaching teens and young adults their birthright of Traditional Ecological/ Indigenous Knowledge will allow them to understand their proving ground, and their journey to adulthood will commence. The internal (female) and external (male) journeys are not exclusive to gender, but are experienced by both, just in different proportions. Rites of passage are taught by Elders through stories, prepared by teaching necessary skills, and tended to by the same gender. Males go out on the land and learn through fasting, self-reliance (almost alone), quick problem solving, physical strength, and stamina. Females go into seclusion and learn through fasting, self-fulfillment (almost alone), focusing on the future, learning patience, restraint, emotional strength, and stamina. Both have elements of calculated pain and suffering. Challenge creates character and inner strength when overcome; rites of passage are a process of creating challenge that has controlled variables.

Being present in a focused state of consciousness can also be understood through the Western concept of meditation, a practice to partake in for a set amount of time. Traditional concepts of meditation are a way of being or Awareness of the universe. Being present, in an observing state, alert and ready to respond, is the opposite of being distracted or preoccupied. Modern thought patterns are out of balance and ego-based. Being present allows thoughts, emotions, and experiences to flow through a person. It requires working through emotions, justice for ill intent, utilizing the experience as learning, and mastering the art of forgiveness. This includes conception, motivation, and execution of intent, or the restraint of acting on impulses.

To have a successful rite of passage, Will generally has to be cultivated. If training of Will was not taught as a child, this leads to difficulties as an adult, as untrained Will can be understood as impulsivity and stubbornness. An incredibly valuable insight in this process of revitalization is the fact that most modern people (Tlingit or other) are not disciplined or trained appropriately to go through fully traditional rites of passage. And the few contemporaries who have undergone the process go through a duration of one week, the traditional version's minimum time span. Most modern people, if not fully immersed in cultural context with preparation, would believe the actual traditional rites are torturous in nature. For this reason, there must be complete understanding of the process and a desire to go through the process by the participant.

The adolescent-to-adulthood transition period is the perfect time to reiterate what a person has learned experientially about their community's perspective of health and wellness, through telling story. This process not only helps to hone a strong, healthy, contributing member of society, it also prepares the young women to make healthy choices for the purpose of bearing strong, healthy, intelligent, spiritually grounded generations to come (DeWitt 2016).

Research Methodology

In order to explore the potential of women's rites of passage for enhancing women's well-being, we decided to create a rite of passage event for healing purposes, which we called the Southeast Women's Rite of Passage (SE WROP) pilot project. We designed the rite of passage event as an applied cultural research project, as well as a healing event, to learn from the experience and apply these lessons in future work. Within the realm of Western research, *applied research* is research that is used to solve practical problems, with the goal of improving the human condition and solving social ills. The main aim of problem-solving research is to find resolutions for the problem in question, reclaiming traditional cultural methods for nurturing the creation of sovereign human beings, and cultivating healthy, thriving communities. The SE WROP pilot project also used qualitative research methods. This subjectivity allows for an ethnographic research approach to focus on the shared attributes, values, norms, practices, language, and material things of the group of people. Because the focus was on translating pre-contact traditions, historical research methods were employed to reflect on and inform the process (Wikibooks 2020), while Indigenous research methods were utilized as the most valuable and applicable set of methods for this project.

Indigenous research brings liberation from the history of oppression and racism, serving to inform the political liberation from struggles of Indigenous Peoples. It is necessary for development, for rebuilding leadership and governance structures, for strengthening social and cultural institutions, for protecting and restoring environments, and for revitalizing language and culture (Smith 2007). The power of Indigenous research is rooted in relationship and reciprocity. Shawn Wilson (2001) describes Indigenous methodology as a means of talking about relational accountability. A researcher answers to all their relations when they are doing research. The methodology must ask different questions. Rather than asking about validity or reliability, it asks, "How am I fulfilling my role or obligation in this relationship?" (Wilson 2001).

Indigenous research Protocols include several ways of approaching the world involving genealogical relations that are layered with reciprocal responsibilities, processes of renewal, and an understanding that humans must be humble toward other beings, entities, and collectives. Scientific inquiry is interwoven with complex genealogical relationships that are at the forefront of each Indigenous people's approach to sustainability. Acting on Protocols that are based on caretaking and stewardship guides scientific inquiry, and plays an integral role in self-determination and revitalizing vibrant ways of life (Whyte, Brewer, and Johnson 2015). Participatory action research is also useful for Indigenous people because it aligns with our axiological beliefs. Action research may have been developed from constructivist or critical theory models, but it fits well into our paradigm because the idea is to improve the reality of people with whom you work (Wilson 2001).

At the time of conception and development of the SE WROP pilot project, the organizer did not realize that using the framework of Tlingit learning systems was, in actuality, the basis for creating Indigenous research methods for Tlingit cultural research. The methods used were as follows: personal experience and understanding, literature reviews, interviews, action participatory groups (Protocols, Ceremony, mentorship, peer teaching, talking circles, cathartic art, storytelling, place-based education), surveys, community presentations and feedback, and informal observation of and check-ins with participants.

Ethnographic interviews, with an informal interview style, were used primarily. The informal interview style is grounded in traditional methods and is defined by cultural norms. Allowing for the natural flow of information through relationship building and storytelling allows the Wisdom Keeper to provide information in the way that they are comfortable with. Formal interview style with an interview schedule and a set list of questions limits capacity, potentially hemming in the interviewer to a set of terminologies or a direction that the Wisdom Keeper may not be familiar with, or limits the opportunity for deep spatial flow of storytelling. Also, of note, due to the over-researched nature of Indigenous communities, questionnaires can immediately change the way the Wisdom Keeper communicates, if at all, and can hinder the flow of information. Just the simple act of writing things down is frowned upon by some Elders, who feel it is an improper way of retaining knowledge, preferring the learner to listen and retain. This way, the identities in association with the content are retained, as it is an important part of establishing legitimacy of the content shared. Stating the Elder's name, cultural affiliation, what they shared, and listing the date and venue are necessary parts in the process of authenticating the knowledge. This accords with appropriate practices for Indigenous methods because the proper identification in association with the content verifies its validity and context.

Participatory action research combines participatory research and action research. *Participatory research* selects issues related to dependence, oppression, and other inequities in need of evaluation. *Action research* uses findings to address community issues. Utilizing both methods involves both the participant and the researchers throughout the process. This method is in congruence with Indigenous research methods because participants are considered experts due to their lived experiences and cultural knowledge. The goal of participatory action research is to influence social change (Watters, Comeau, and Restall 2010).

Participants were chosen based on their cultural affiliation, life experiences, service to community and culture, general age range, desire to make a difference in their communities, and capacity to commit to the project. Peer educators were chosen for their cultural affiliation and area of expertise. Female Elder mentors were chosen based on their level of contribution to the content of the project, capacity to attend/mobility, and their desire to attend. Local female Elder mentors were chosen for their culturally relevant role as representatives of the Clan whose traditional territory the SE WROP was being held on. The camp cook was chosen based on culinary skills to create and provide a specialized menu, cultural affiliation, gender, and age. Male Elder guest speakers were chosen for their cultural affiliation, cultural knowledge, and positive reputations within the cultural group.

During the pilot project, the methods used were cultural Protocols, Ceremony, mentorship, peer teaching, seclusion, talking circles, storytelling, journaling, cathartic art, and place-based education. The participants were instructed to create family trees before coming to the pilot project if they did not already know their family, Clan, moiety, house, or village lineage. This was an integral part of understanding how the participants were in relationship with each other and what Protocols or relationship functions they served to their peers.

Surveys were filled out during the pilot project and after the participants returned home. This was to understand what they were going through at the time and to gather the qualitative interpretations of the participant's experience. The questions were modelled on how they felt personally about the experience, what benefits they believed it would have for their community, and how they would like to see it manifest in the future. The event coordinators and participants signed media and content release forms giving permission to use the qualitative data gathered for presentation and further works.

Community Engagement and Feedback

The purpose, process, and outcomes were presented at the Southeast Clan Conference held in Sitka in 2013, and then presented again at the Alaska Native Studies Conference held at the University of Alaska, Anchorage, in 2013. Community involvement is an integral part of Indigenous research methodology. Through engaging the community and inviting feedback from community members, the researchers and the community are immersed in a relational process of research and development. With the history of exploitation, research on or about Indigenous people was written about in an objective manner, creating superficial understanding and relegating community members as irrelevant. From the Indigenous research framework, community engagement and feedback is not only integral to the process, it is fundamental to upholding minimal ethical standards, especially cultural Protocols.

Once the presentations were given, the community members were invited to give their feedback on the project and information, and this feedback was then integrated into the findings. While informing the community is a necessary step, involving the community in the formation of research and programs that affect them is a valuable aspect of encouraging self-determination.

Indirect observations, through maintaining interpersonal relationships, have been made in regard to the participants' growth as influenced by their experiences and participation in the pilot project. While the participants were of the same cultural group, they were and are geographically separated by vast distances, rugged terrain, and limited transportation options. The different social connections and interactions that have been maintained by the group since the pilot project occurred have been observed through various forms of communication, including, but not limited to, in-person dialogue, electronic mail, social media (direct and indirect), telephonically, and through Indigenous forms of observations made through social networks. To be fully immersed in the process, by becoming part of the participant cohort, I was exposed to information that would not have otherwise been accessible. The immersion process includes following Protocols that are core to the culture, giving an acquaintance and intimacy that cannot be gained any other way. Trust is a factor in successful outcomes, and is fundamental in establishing social currency, which is a necessary process for becoming a successful Indigenous researcher and will provide more support and success to the final project or program.

Indigenous research methods are rooted firmly in the Protocols of the researcher and the research participant's intersectionality of shared culture and heritage. The researcher's community and culture's beliefs, spirituality, and relationality are part of the research—with the engagement of spiritual beliefs, ancestors, oral story, traditional lands, family, community, and all our relations (birds, plants, animals, fish, insects, unseen, and in-between) as co-collaborators (personal communication with Kyle P. Whyte, 2017). Indigenous research methods are the best way to conduct research that is holistic in scope, and that serves the purpose of repairing culture and reclaiming Traditional Knowledge and practices. This positions the researcher in their own process and creativity, making the researcher a cultural Wisdom Keeper who will then be responsible for the intergenerational transference of knowledge gained through the research. With this understanding of Indigenous research, it can be said that the Tlingit people were all taught to be researchers as the function of basic education and identity of being Tlingit.

Indigenous people need to do Indigenous research because we have lifelong learning and relationships as well. Research is not just something that is out there: it is something you are building for yourself and for your community (Wilson 2001).

Overview of the Southeast Women's Rite of Passage Project

Traditional interviews and advisement sessions with Alaska Native Elders were started over one year before the SE WROP pilot project was held. Planning, literature review, and garnering funding all happened simultaneously during the one-year period. Process and Protocols were mapped out, and the two forms of research were used to identify the types of knowledge, activities, and participants that would be engaged in the process.

The Women's Rite of Passage involved Elder advisors Rosa Miller, Naa Tlaa Thleenaidee; Anna J. Schoppert, Naa Tlaa Ishkitaan; Della Cheney, Naa Tlaa Katch.adi; and Charlette Silverly; and Honorary Aunties Suzi Williams, Tlingit traditional weaver; and Barbara Franks, Alaska Native Tribal Health Consortium (ANTHC) program associate Behavioral Health Services. The participant educators who stayed for the duration of the week were Vivian Mork, Wrangell/Tlingit traditions keeper/ language teacher; Alex McKenna, Teslin Traditional Council; Liz Medicine Crow, Elder-in-training interim director First Alaskan's Institute; Tanya Bitonti, City Council, School Board, XKKF tribal nonprofit, Haida Corporation; Renae Mathson, diabetes educator, Southeast Alaska Regional Health Consortium; Meda DeWitt, TH, ANTHC program associate Health Promotion Disease Prevention; Flora Deacon,

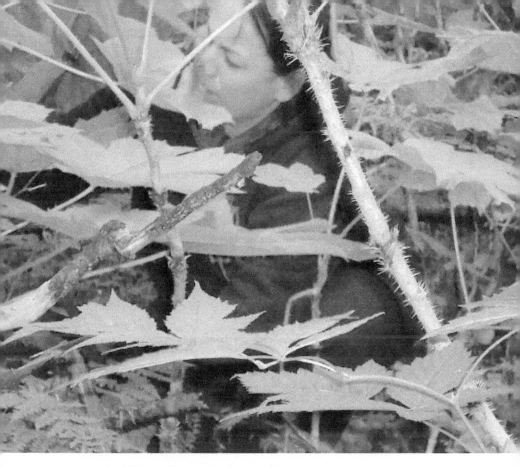

FIGURE 8.1 *Alex McKenna, Tlingit, Teslin Traditional Council, harvesting devil's club. [Photo by Meda DeWitt.]*

camp chef, rural nutrition services educator, University of Alaska, Fairbanks, featured chef TFCC; and Margaret Hoffman David, BS, ANTHC program manager Health Promotion Disease Prevention. We also had the following guest speakers and visiting educators who stayed for less then one day: Taija Revels, Epi STD/STI educator ANTHC; Desiree Bergeron, registered dietician, ANTHC program manager Nutrition and Traditional Foods; Barbara Franks, ANTHC program associate Behavioral Health Services on Men's Roles; David Katzeek, Shangukeidi Lingit language educator and storyteller; David Kanosh, Deisheetaan healer and Clan leader; and Walter Porter, Alaska Native mythologist, Tlingit legends keeper, Elder and mentor from Yakutat, Alaska.

The event was held at Juneau Methodist Camp at mile 28 "out the road," and was supported by multiple funders.[5]

The first day was about getting settled in and making proper introductions. Traditional introductions commenced, as well as contemporary facilitation methods such as ice breakers were incorporated. The group created agreements regarding their expectations of themselves and each other's conduct. Discussions about Protocol and structure of conduct during menses, and an overview of the educational sections, were presented: nutrition, self-care, daily meditation, activities, cultural learning, sacred teachings, Lingít language immersion, cultural Shkalneek/Tlaagú (stories/legends).

Safety was reviewed, along with distribution of whistles and flashlights, and journals were handed out along with "self-scratchers." The Tlingit people incorporated personal scratching devices. Scratchers had dual purposes: one function was the reduction of infection from breaking the skin with dirty nails, and the other was to be mindful of not excessively scratching or picking at oneself—a sign of lack of discipline.

The successive days included a morning prayer and smudging, a movement session, meals, and instructions on selected topics. During the gathering, a specific menu was provided based on vegetarian, organic, dairy/gluten-free, low sugar, and no artificial colours, flavours, or fragrances. The only animal protein that was provided was salmon that was caught in a net, not by a hook. No stimulants or altering substances were allowed—this included coffee and cigarettes. Each day included a seclusion session that progressively grew in duration throughout the gathering.

FIGURE 8.2 *(opposite)*
Specific foods were made in accordance to a modified fasting process.
The women also abstained from coffee, sugar, meat, and processed foods.
[Photos by Meda DeWitt.]

FIGURE 8.2A *(top) Blueberries, strawberries, and nasturtium flowers.*

FIGURE 8.2B *(centre) Salad of raw vegetables.*

FIGURE 8.2C *(bottom) Salad of raw greens with pine nuts.*

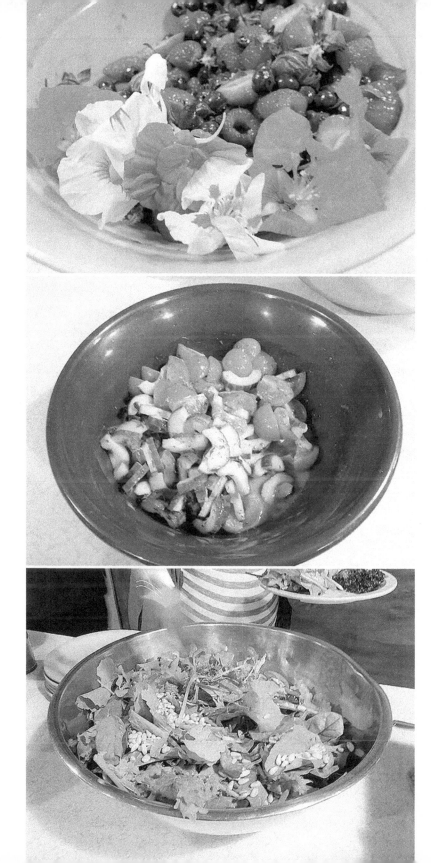

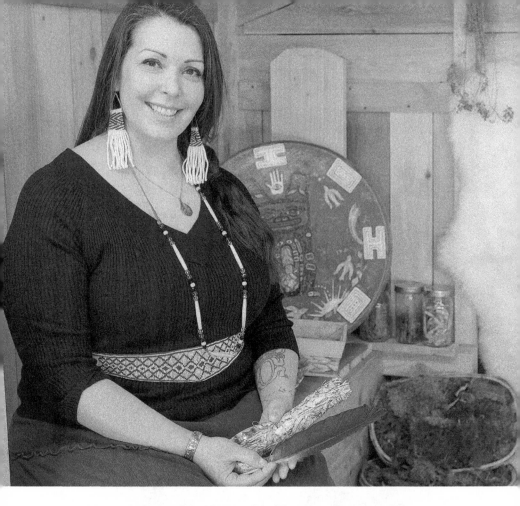

FIGURE 8.3 *Meda DeWitt, Tśa Tsée Náakw/Khaat kła.at, Naanyaa.aayí Clan, presenting a talk on the woman's house and women's rites of passage at the Anchorage Museum in September 2020. Used with permission of the Anchorage Museum.*

Education topics included Ceremony, steam bath, seclusion, Tlingit language, plants, prenatal/post-natal self- and child care and the fourth trimester, Elder women's teachings, Tlingit women standing in their traditional roles as leaders, weaving, life planning and autonomy, traditional food/nutrition, sex education, domestic violence, crafts involving traditional materials such as devil's club medicine sticks, and men in the Tlingit culture's traditional and contemporary roles.

We reflected on the program as it unfolded and identified various ways that the event could have been even more effective. We felt that we could interview the speakers more in-depth to gain a better understanding of intentions, and have all the educators, facilitators, and Elders (if possible) be together the entire time. Less in and out is desirable, as it causes less disruption. In the future we should go before the event to review different locations for cleanliness, access, seclusion, use, and feel. We should also invite an Auntie, Grandma, Mother, or female mentor to come with the participants. Emotional Freedom Technique (EFT) training and traditional self-healing methods would be beneficial as part of the tools people are taught. When finally adding youth, we must be prepared to add a background check process for adults to ensure safety and a good process. We need to make seclusion, sweat, and other Protocols more of a priority. We also need to refine the health education to three main topics and should visit different aspects of these topics. Finally, we need to make sure the hands-on portions are included, and have backup educators in case one does not show up.

More than one gathering for a group is important. This is a process of change, and integration does not happen magically overnight or over one week. This is a profound topic, and people are calling for this kind of change, and the movement will grow. The biggest trigger was child sexual abuse, and was the only topic that presented a challenge. One of the presenters did not discuss the topic in a way that was trauma-informed and triggered one of the participants. The Elder women handled the situation in a traditional format. Discussion of healing from child sexual assault in a trauma-informed way needs to be taught, along with training on how to assist in community healing and justice.

Traditionally, women on their menses or during their rites of passage would not gather or process plants. Even though I explained this to every participant, they still wanted to learn and work with plants. Even our Elder Rosa Miller was more focused on plants. After a couple of days, I just surrendered to our Elder women's guidance, and we harvested/processed some devil's club and nagoon berries. I realized that what we are craving is the connection to Mother Earth/Nature. We yearn for that wisdom that used to be commonplace, our birthright. The connection to Mother Earth is a major component of rites of passage and being a woman, therefore skills building around the area of wild foods/medicines is fundamentally important and can stand alone or in collaboration with Western health education.

All the women (except one) were/are interested in fully traditional rites of passage with weeklong seclusion, sweat, fasting, and so on.

Participant Pre-Evaluation

We engaged in a participant pre-evaluation for the ANTHC SE WROP 2012 pilot project. The following discussion will enumerate the questions of the pre-evaluation and the responses we received, paraphrased to retain coherence.

1) *What are your personal expectations out of WROP: SE 2012 pilot project?*
The participants came to learn and gain an understanding of their traditions and culture. They showed a deep interest in contributing to the process, as well as taking back the teachings to their communities to improve the health of their communities.

2) *How do you believe that WROP: SE protocol 2012 pilot project can benefit the Alaskan Native Peoples?*
The participants believe that rites of passage are necessary steps in the process of becoming a whole person without becoming stuck in life stages. Rites of passage will allow Alaska Native Peoples to move beyond the pain into the light, giving Native women/people a better understanding of self-worth. By teaching each other our traditions and meanings of culture, an understanding and a sense of belonging will occur. Every culture should have a wonderful opportunity like this—it is important to empower Alaska Native women through traditional lenses to prevent and combat social ills, which will affect our families in a positive way at their core.

By creating a template for other cultural groups so it's workable and supportive of their culture's prerogatives, we will be using our experiences to help seed Native healthy communities. "If it was good enough for our Ancestors, it's good enough for us."

Participant Post-Evaluation

We also engaged in a post-project evaluation, which I summarize below with both exact quotes and paraphrased to retain coherence.

1) *How did this event compare to your personal expectations of WROP: SE protocol 2012 pilot project?*

Overall, the women expressed that it was a learning experience, and the development of women's rites of passage is important. Some of them questioned the amount or age of the participants, but "quickly learned the size we had was just right." For some, the event went above and beyond their personal expectations, citing that the hands-on and listening to the Elders'/speakers' components were eye-opening experiences.

- "Gave me a clear understanding of what the rites of passage are and why it is so important in our culture."
- "I will never forget how important rites of passage were to our people."
- "What I've learned from all whom attended, this knowledge will benefit my community for years to come."
- "I am blessed to have been a part of this program."

2) *How do you believe that WROP: SE protocol can benefit the Alaskan Native Peoples?*

- "WROP is very important to the survival of AK Native Peoples. It will help us heal who we are at our core which will help to prevent and combat not only chronic diseases but also social ills such as suicide."
- "The benefits could be profound, our culture needs to be ingrained in the mainstream of consciousness, from birth to death, making ceremony is an anchor for vessels of wisdom—our women."
- "Give them an identity of who they are."
- "I believe that this can benefit the entire world; however, for Alaska Native People it's an empowering tool that will help rebuild self-esteem in our young ones—making healthy adults."

- "Through ceremony will healing begin."
- "They may be comfortable with who they are."
- "Super important for a whole and well-being. We can learn from SE structure how to piece together WROP in other regions."
- "Yes—I believe that this program would benefit all Alaskan Native People. It would give many natives a clear understanding of who they are and for many a feeling of self-worth."
- "By serving as a flexible template/curriculum guide for all our Native cultural groups in Alaska to adapt to their cultural needs and ways, we can help ensure our Girls/Women know how to take care of themselves physically, spiritually, mentally/intellectually, and emotionally. This will make us stronger, healthier, and more able to thrive as a collective group of Native peoples and as individuals who can help ensure our cultures are protected and strengthened, while at the same time our health/wellness continues to improve as a community, as relatives, and as individuals. By improving the strength of our women and our cultures, we improve all other factors of our lives—our kids, our men, our cultures/languages, our lands, our access and use of foods and medicines, our villages, and organizations, etc."

3) What suggestions do you have for the improvement of the WROP: SE protocol?

- "It would be important to have the core group meet again and bring Elder women who have been influential in their lives to continue expanding and solidifying a cohesive adaptable curriculum."
- "Perhaps start a 'talking circle' on the issues in each community—sending teams of previous participants to—jump start."
- "Perhaps record men with digital storytelling tools. Starting the conversation on Men's ROP."
- "Let's go back to our communities and research, then do, and then come together 1 yr. from now to see what results we have created."
- "How can one improve on perfection?"
- "Place equal participation on each person."
- "A planning committee."

- "I believe WROP should have their own camp with many of the traditional ways of life being incorporated into the map like the cedar curtains for seclusion also a main sweat area—but also option to build your own. I believe the women did a great job keeping it very traditional and it was a wonderful life changing experience."
- "Do more of them and add in more cultural foods and activities as we continue to build it up, and help folks understand how to apply it in their everyday, moving from talking to walking. Build in understanding about land stewardship and Clan ownership concepts, etc...and the role of women in those areas. Help group members identify the big goals then create activities to flesh our ROP more, capture all this vital information. I think this was done a bit, I just think it is a growth area rather than 'improvement.' Does that make sense?"
- "It was an honor and a privilege to participate; strong women are beautiful."

Conclusions

Rites of passage are one of the tools for rebuilding culture, as they are foundational in the process of building healthy people and strong communities. Rites of passage do not stand alone but function as a capstone of learning how to be a Tlingit and understanding the Tlingit way of life. Much like climbing a staircase of personal growth, a rite of passage is the landing before the ascent of the next flight. There are many people who are stuck because they did not receive the proper building blocks to move to the next level. They are stuck in a cycle of revisiting the neglected lessons that lead to the deficit in personal growth (Erikson and Erikson 1997), thus never really entering into adulthood (Campbell 1949).

Indigenous people from around the world are calling for rites of passage for men and women. They are an identified part of human development that is lacking or that have been replaced by Western constructs (some of which are extremely negative), such as menses being viewed as a curse or unclean. Sixteen years old is old enough to drive a car and gain independence, a seventeen-year-old can watch R-rated movies, at eighteen a person is an adult and can buy tobacco, at twenty-one years old you can purchase alcohol and drink

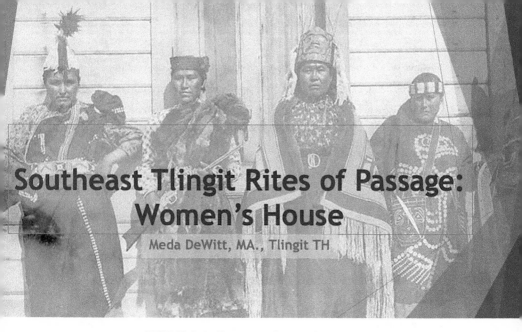

Southeast Tlingit Rites of Passage: Women's House

Meda DeWitt, MA., Tlingit TH

FIGURE 8.4 *SE WROP Senior Presentation Program Cover, 2017.*

in establishments, thirty years old is the age of moving into real adulthood, and at fifty you are over the hill. In contrast, the act of deep self-control practised in long durations, lasting anywhere from one week up to one year, allows the individual to know who they were without the daily influences of others. When they emerge from their training, they can be expected to have inner and outer discipline of self, living and operating from a fully present state of being. As a good friend once said, "They were taught how to own their own skin."

The women in the Tlingit culture are the well of wisdom that spans back through all the women before them from time immemorial. It was their duty to preserve the songs, dances, stories, skills, and understanding of what it was to be Tlingit in the most rooted sense. The Naa Tláa (head woman of a Clan) and Elder women were looked to as a guide to the Chieftains of the Tlingit people. They were expected to keep balance within the Tlingit culture as an integral part of society; they transmitted knowledge and wisdom to the younger generations about how to be a real human being, and how to be Tlingit for the continuation of a living culture. In this process, energy is focused inwards on themselves, searching out what they want to be when they grow up, what values they uphold, and what they want to accomplish in this lifetime. It is also a time of spiritual communion with the ancestors and the creator, receiving guidance.

Through traditional rites of passage, the community cultivates the time, space, and process to grow. The act of being in seclusion creates a stronger connection to themselves, their culture, the community, and Earth, formulating and solidifying their identity as a Tlingit person. It gives time to introspect and meditate on who they want to be and where they are going (Cheney 2007). Combining traditional activities, education on best health practices, and creating strong social ties to mentors and support systems in the community allows an individual to access the building blocks that guide transition into their next level of growth.

NOTES

1. *Baasee', quyana,* and *quyaana* all mean "thank you" in Koyukon, Yup'ik, and Iñupiaq, respectively.

2. von Langsdorff visited Sitka, Alaska, in 1805–1806.

3. According to Mann and Peteet (1994), the Last Glacial Maximum in southeast Alaska was from 23,000 BP (before the present) to around 14,700 BP. Climatic turbulence characterized the deglaciation period in Alaska, and the retreat of glaciers to within their Holocene footprints seems to have taken place by about 11,000 years ago (see Briner et al. 2017). There were also Holocene glacial re-advances in this dynamic region. Cruikshank's book dates stories to the Little Ice Age, which is a period of historic glacial advance between the years 1550 to 1850.

4. Personal communication with Dr. Ann Bullock, 2016, University of Alaska, Anchorage, Alaska Trust Training Cooperative.

5. Funders included ANTHC Wellness Division, Health Promotion Disease Prevention–Funding, ANTHC Behavioral Health Services, Suicide Prevention–Funding, ANTHC Behavioral Health Services, Domestic Violence Prevention–Funding, ANTHC Behavioral Health Services, Substance Abuse Prevention–Funding, First Alaskan's Institute-sponsored Employee, SEARHC Health Promotion Disease Prevention, Diabetes-sponsored Employee, and Teslin Tlingit Council-sponsored Employee.

REFERENCES

Brave Heart, M.Y.H., J. Chase, J. Etkins, and D.B. Altschul. 2011. "Historical Trauma among
Indigenous Peoples of the Americas: Concepts, Research, and Clinical Considerations."
Journal of Psychoactive Drugs 43, no. 4: 282–90. https://pubmed.ncbi.nlm.nih.
gov/22400458/.

Briner, P., J.P. Tulenko, D.S. Kaufman, N.E. Young, J.F. Baichtal, and A. Lesnek. 2017. "The
Last Deglaciation of Alaska." *Cuadernos de Investigacion Geografica* 43, no. 2: 429–48.
http://doi.org/10.18172/cig.3229.

Campbell, J. 1949. *The Hero with a Thousand Faces.* 1st Edition, Bollingen Foundation.
New York: Pantheon Press.

Cheney, L. 2007. "On Becoming a Mother." *Making Birth Safe in the US* (blog). February 17,
2007. http://hospitalbirthdebate.blogspot.com/2007/02/more-about-tlingit-and-birth.html.

Cruikshank, J. 2005. *Do Glaciers Listen? Local Knowledge, Colonial Encounters, and Social
Imagination.* Vancouver: UBC Press.

Cruikshank, J. 2001. "Glaciers and Climate Change: Perspectives from Oral Tradition." *Arctic*
54, no. 4: 377–93.

Dauenhauer, N., and R. Dauenhauer. 1987. *Haa Shuká, Our Ancestors: Tlingit Oral
Narratives.* Seattle: University of Washington Press.

DeWitt, M. 2016. "Teens Healing from Trauma and Traditional Healing." Lecture presented
at Nenana School District, Nenana, AK, August 19, 2016.

DeWitt, M. 2015. "Traditional Health Based Practices." Course curriculum, Center for Human
Development, University of Alaska, Anchorage.

Dong, M., W.H. Giles, V.J. Felitti, S.R. Dube, J.E. Williams, D.P. Chapman, and R.F. Anda.
2004. "Insights into Causal Pathways for Ischemic Heart Disease: Adverse Childhood
Experiences Study." *Circulation* 110, no. 13: 1761–66. https://doi.org/10.1161/01.
CIR.0000143074.54995.7F.

Emmons, G.T. (1911) 1991. *The Tlingit Indians.* Edited by F. de Laguna. Seattle: University of
Washington Press.

Erikson, E.H., and J.M. Erikson. 1997. *The Life Cycle Completed.* New York: W.W. Norton.

Felitti, V.J., R.F. Anda, D. Nordenberg, D.F. Williamson, A.M. Spitz, V. Edwards, M.P. Koss,
and J.S. Marks. 1998. "Relationship of Childhood Abuse and Household Dysfunction to
Many of the Leading Causes of Death in Adults: The Adverse Childhood Experiences
(ACE) Study." *American Journal of Preventive Medicine* 14, no. 4: 245–58. https://doi.
org/10.1016/S0749-3797(98)00017-8.

Holmberg, H.J. 1855. *Ethnographische Skizzen über die Völker des Russischen Amerikas.*
Vol 1. *Die Thlinkitchen.Siw Konjagen.* Acta Sicietate Scientificae Fennicae 4.
Hesingfors. [Translation of quoted passage by Frederica de Laguna.]

Jonaitis, A. 1988. "Women, Marriage, Mouths and Feasting: The Symbolism of Tlingit Labrets." In *Marks of Civilization*, edited by A. Rubin, 191–208. Los Angeles: Museum of Cultural History—UCLA.

Krause, A. 1972. *The Tlingit Indians: Results of a Trip to Northwest Coast of America and the Bering Straits*. Translated by E. Gunther. Seattle: University of Washington Press.

La Salle, M. 2013/2014. "Labrets and Their Social Context in Coastal British Columbia." *BC Studies* 180 (Winter): 123–53.

Langsdorff, G.H. 1814. *Voyages and Travels in Various Parts of the World during the Years 1803, 1804, 1805, 1806 and 1807*. Vol. 2. London: Henry Colburn.

Lines, L.-A., and C.G. Jardine. 2019. "Connection to the Land as a Youth-Identified Social Determinant of Indigenous Peoples' Health." *BMC Public Health* 19, no. 176. https://doi.org/10.1186/s12889-018-6383-8.

Mann, D.H., and D.M. Peteet. 1994. "Extent and Timing of the Last Glacial Maximum in Southwestern Alaska." *Quaternary Research* 42, no. 2: 136–48. https://doi.org/10.1006/qres.1994.1063.

Reddish, J. 2013. "Labrets: Piercing and Stretching on the Northwest Coast and in Amazonia." *Mundo Amazonico* 4: 57–75.

Smith, L.T. 2007. "On Tricky Ground: Researching the Native in the Age of Uncertainty." In *The Landscape of Qualitative Research*, edited by N.K. Denzin and Y.S. Lincoln, 113–43. Los Angeles: SAGE Publications.

Stoppler, M. n.d. "Endorphins: Natural Pain and Stress Fighters." *MedicineNet*. http://www.medicinenet.com/script/main/art.asp?articlekey=55001.

Turner, N. 1979. *Plants in British Columbia Indian Technology*. Victoria: British Columbia Provincial Museum.

Veniaminof, I. (1840) 1984. *Notes on the Islands of the Unalaska District*. Kingston, ON: Limestone Press.

Watters, J., S. Comeau, and G. Restall. 2010. *Participatory Action Research: An Education Tool for Citizen-Users of Community Mental Health Services*. University of Manitoba. http://umanitoba.ca/rehabsciences/media/par_manual.pdf.

Wikibooks. 2020. "Research Methods/Types of Research." https://en.wikibooks.org/wiki/Research_Methods/Types_of_Research.

Wilson, S. 2001. "What Is an Indigenous Research Methodology?" *Canadian Journal of Native Education* 25, no. 2: 175–79.

Whyte, K.P., J.P. Brewer, and J.T. Johnson. 2015. "Weaving Indigenous Science, Protocols and Sustainability Science." *Sustainability Science* 11: 25–32. https://doi.org/10.1007/s11625-015-0296-6.

9 Health and Healing on the Edges of Canada

A Photovoice Project in Ulukhaktok, NT

DOROTHY BADRY AND ANNIE I. GOOSE

Dorothy Badry is a professor in the Faculty of Social Work at the University of Calgary, and Annie Goose is an Inuvialuit Elder, language expert, and craftsperson from Ulukhaktok, NT. They collaborated on the Brightening Our Home Fires project to address women's health and FASD (Fetal Alcohol Spectrum Disorder) prevention, which took place in four communities in the Northwest Territories, including Yellowknife, Łutselk'e, Behchokǫ̀, and Ulukhaktok (2011–2012), using the Photovoice methodology described below. The chapter included here is based on their collaborative research project report and was revised for inclusion in this book.

My Family—Enjoying the Simple Things in Life

My bonding with them is more genuine than ever before. And we are the best of friends, my boys and my daughters. We can share, and laugh and be real with each other. That gave me great inspiration to carry on with my own life. Photovoice is a very safe passage for one to express themselves. Our words and pictures convey more about our inner being and support healing more than I realized. Taking pictures can reflect everyday reality and contribute to healing your inner being. This experiencing gives you an enjoyment—just being true to yourself and those around you. There are moments that you

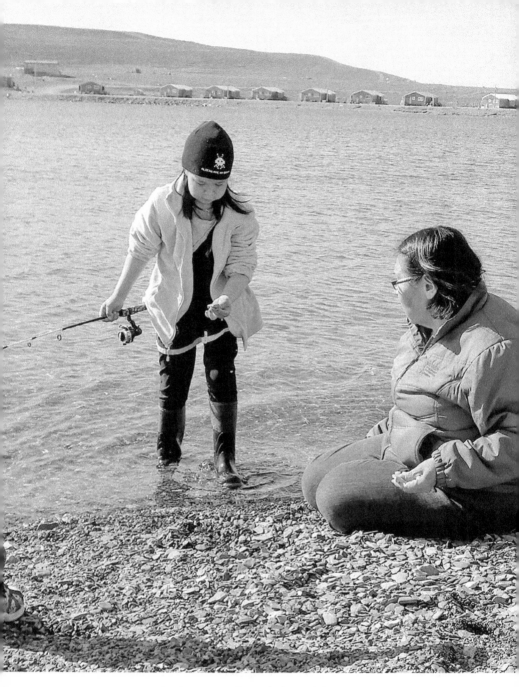

FIGURE 9.1 *My family—enjoying the simple things of life.*

never realize you see until you take a picture and then you see it—differently. Photovoice through images and true colours offers inner peace and enjoyment of moments in your life that you never thought were important.

— PHOTO BY ANNIE GOOSE, Ulukhaktok, NT, June 26, 2012

Introduction

We begin this chapter with the above photo and Annie's commentary in order to identify and illustrate the powerful reflections offered through Photovoice—the guiding methodology for this research. Photovoice is a qualitative research methodology used in community-based and health research as a method to document local experiences and realities as seen through the eyes of the participant taking photographs. Photovoice is a powerful methodology to use in reflecting the lived experience of people in community. Wang and Burris (1997) identify Photovoice as a feminist method that involves taking photographs that reflect lived experience within a community in relation to issues or concerns, and, as such, it offers a place to engage in critical dialogues and supports sharing the information gathered with policy makers.

The cameras are something that are useful for daily living, taking family photos and today social media has a lot of photos out there. I think the most powerful way of expressing self—it shows in individuals showing photos of what is important to them—whether be family, children, the land, community events, hunting, fishing and traditional cultural activities. Cultural vibrancy is shown in many ways in the photos.

— ANNIE GOOSE, Ulukhaktok, NT, December 5, 2012

Further discussion of the Photovoice methodology takes place in the section on methodology below.

How do you open a dialogue on the complex health topic of FASD prevention in northern and remote communities that is sensitively grounded from a trauma-informed perspective? This question cannot be addressed without considering the historical impact of contact with outsiders and the legacy of colonial impact on the North. Communities on the northern edges of Canada continue to grow and develop, and family life is deeply valued. The northern environment, while often cold and harsh, is culturally rich. We know contextually that women face many challenges in the North. Health care, safety and security in cases of domestic violence, poverty, substance abuse, and homelessness are all problems that pose risk in small, remote communities. Other challenges for remote communities include timely access to treatment, and often having to travel long distances to access health care or addictions treatment. There is bleakness in the winter, and concerns about substance use rise while suicidal thoughts simmer, when darkness descends 24/7. The winter months are often challenging in small, remote, northern communities, and illness and deaths among community members are deeply felt. Health promotion is an important focus of Beaufort-Delta Health and Social Services and includes support for chronic disease, Elder supports, prenatal and post-natal care, and disease prevention, and provides access to regional health services, including dental care, diabetes education, nutrition, and other allied supports as identified by Ulukhaktok Health Services.

A project was undertaken in the Northwest Territories between 2010 and 2012 called Brightening Our Home Fires. Members of the Canada FASD Research Network Action Team on Women's Health (2010) initiated the research and engaged with four communities. The financial contribution of the First Nations & Inuit Health Branch supported this research project. The focus of this chapter is on the work completed in the community of Ulukhaktok, above the Arctic Circle and located on Victoria Island.

Ulukhaktok is a small hamlet with a population of over four hundred people, and is a remote community on the Beaufort Sea that is only accessible by airplane most of the year. There were twelve women involved in this project, and co-author Annie Goose from Ulukhaktok was a research facilitator and translator for the project. Annie also participated in the Photovoice work and shared deep insights into health and healing, and her reflections of this experience are included in this chapter. The purpose of the Brightening Our Home Fires project was to understand factors women see as important in health and healing in the North and to consider protective and supportive of women's health.

We recognize that FASD prevention and discussions about addictions are deeply personal topics and not something that women would want to talk about in front of others. We also acknowledge that there are limitations to this research. Asking directly about FASD poses a barrier to working with women in the North. While some awareness of FASD exists, there is no infrastructure in small remote communities for diagnosis. It is also recognized that it is a challenge to identify the cause of a disability, due to the stigma associated with alcohol use and pregnancy. It is important that individuals with disabilities are integrated and included as members of the community, and it is important in remote communities to provide natural supports wherever possible.

This chapter will focus on the value of Photovoice as a means to talk about complex health concerns, using an approach that is nonthreatening and is grounded in imagery and text. We discovered that using Photovoice diminishes perceived stigma, fear, and apprehension in relation to talking about FASD as a health concern, and our conversations focused on health— not FASD. Strong themes emerging from this research included the healing nature of family connections, culture, and community. We will report the major themes of the research, share some images, and reflect on the process. As co-authors of this chapter, we collaborated to provide some contextual information about health and social concerns in the North, while balancing these issues with insight and lived experience that is grounded in culture and community.

Setting the Stage for FASD Prevention: Review of the Literature

The topic of women's health and healing in relation to addictions and FASD prevention is a critical, yet daunting, topic. The Ajunnginiq Centre, National Aboriginal Health Organization (2006) undertook an environmental scan of service and gaps in relation to FASD. Its report documented efforts being undertaken since 2003 in relation to developing awareness materials, and holding community-based workshops with an overall focus on prevention. Prevention efforts have included sharing information across regions and work conducted with the Canadian Prenatal Nutrition Program, which has been very active in the Arctic regions of Canada. It is difficult to acknowledge that a child may be having difficulties due to alcohol exposure during pregnancy due to stigma, and it was suggested that community voices, especially Elders, aid in contributing to discussions on prevention. The other challenge is a lack of specialized health care services in remote and isolated communities, which often requires extensive travel for health care treatment (Pauktuutit Inuit Women of Canada 2010). If a concern is identified that FASD may be an issue for a child, it would take substantial effort to access diagnostic resources, and communities often have more pressing concerns, such as poverty and a lack of adequate housing.

The Northwest Territories Child and Family Services Act is the guiding legislation that outlines the circumstances and conditions under which Child and Family Services could become involved. Involvement with child welfare can also be stigmatizing in the North, particularly in small communities in contrast to larger urban centres. In relation to child welfare involvement, Northwest Territories Health and Social Services (2011) reported,

> Children may receive services because they were abused or neglected. Other children may come into care voluntarily and/or receive services because they have unmanageable behavioral problems resulting from developmental delays, mental health issues or Fetal Alcohol Spectrum Disorder (FASD). (70)

In the 2013–2014 *Annual Report of the Director of Child and Family Services* (Government of the Northwest Territories 2014–2015), section 7(3) (g) of the act identifies the concern that children with mental or emotional health problems, or other developmental conditions (disabilities), may be in need of support or intervention if families cannot access services, or are unable for a number of reasons to engage with such services. Society places the responsibility to protect and nurture children with biological parents or extended family members. Child protection agencies, while responsible for investigating allegations of neglect/child abuse, can also be an avenue to offer and provide supports to families through voluntary agreements to ensure the safety and well-being of children. There are limited resources in small communities, and children with disabilities are generally integrated into existing programs within schools. It is not uncommon in the Northwest Territories for children to live with extended family, and this is an important aspect of the social fabric of remote communities.

The *Annual Report of the Director of Child and Family Services* (Government of the Northwest Territories 2015–2016) reported that approximately one thousand children receive some form of service either through agreement with the family (66.4 per cent), or by court order (33.6 per cent). The use of voluntary agreements is reported as a means to support and strengthen families and is consistently used with families, as well as with youth ages sixteen to eighteen needing supports that include housing, financial aid, and support with treatment for addictions. Further, rates of children in permanent care have declined from 252 in 2006–2007 to 167 as of 2016. A primary concern in the Northwest Territories is parents with drug, alcohol, or solvent problems, and this is a major concern in referrals to Child and Family Services. This concern was reiterated in the 2013–2014 report of the director of Child and Family Services, and the need to address alcohol use and its impact on families remains a focus. It was indicated that there are fifteen Healthy Family Programs in the Northwest Territories. Further, this report suggests that the need exists to differentiate between cases of child neglect and child abuse. From a social determinant of health perspective, this is an important consideration, which leaves room for recognizing that poverty and inadequate housing are often contributing factors to children requiring intervention or support. *Building Stronger Families: An Action Plan to Transform Child and Family Services* (Northwest Territories Health and Social Services 2014) and the adoption of a structured decision-making model are key tools in child protective services to support the goal of building stronger families. New directions have been undertaken in the Northwest Territories focused on the *Building Stronger Families* action plan.

The *Report on Substance Use and Addiction* (Northwest Territories Health and Social Services 2015) reported that the impact of addictions is deeply felt in families and communities, and includes the use of 2012 data on addiction, including alcohol, tobacco, drugs, and gambling. It was noted that children of residential school survivors were at much higher risk of alcohol addiction compared to those whose parents did not have this experience. For example, "Of those who reported a parent had gone to residential school, 25% are considered heavy infrequent drinkers, compared to 16% of those who did not have a parent attend" (Northwest Territories Health and Social Services 2015, 37). Additionally, alcohol-related harms were reported to be much higher for individuals living in small communities, often impacting social cohesion in smaller communities. The same report indicates that 75 per cent (Aboriginal and non-Aboriginal) of the population that consumed alcohol are current drinkers, of whom 84 per cent were within the 25–39 age range, 74 per cent (15–24), 72 per cent (40–59), and 59 per cent (60 and older) (Northwest Territories Health and Social Services 2015, 9).

The government released the Mental Wellness and Addictions Recovery Action Plan in 2019, and it calls for the need to reduce stigma around addictions and mental health to increase supportive pathways for addiction recovery, to provide more coordinated and integrated services that recognize family at the centre of recovery, and to strengthen community-based supports, aftercare, and peer support for individuals with mental health and addiction problems. In this action plan, pathways to health have been developed with a focus on increased access to services that address mental health and addictions. The plan recognizes that there are many paths to addiction recovery.

The Social Determinants of Health are social factors contributing to the attainment of a complete state of physical and mental well-being (World Health Organization 2008). Health is impacted by social and economic factors such as income, wealth distribution, employment, education, and by the working and living conditions experienced by different populations and communities. The social determinants of health do not exist in isolation to each other; they are intertwined and inevitably affect quality of life. Access to the basics in life such as food, shelter and clothing, and health and social care are intended to be universally available to all citizens in Canada. The social determinants of health are critical to examine in relation to FASD prevention, as social and economic factors include income, wealth distribution, employment, education, and living conditions. Employment is a major challenge in northern, remote communities as so few jobs exist in small hamlets. Cameron

(2011) compiled a list of social determinants of health as they relate to the northern reality and context, which include acculturation, productivity, income distribution, housing, education, food security, health care services, social safety nets, quality of early life, addictions, and the environment.

In a newer report, Inuit Tapiriit Kanatami (ITK) (2014) quote the World Health Organization (2013) in defining social determinants of health as "the conditions in which people are born, grow, live, work and age, including the health system. These circumstances are shaped by the distribution of money, power and resources at global, national and local levels, which are themselves influenced by policy choices" (3). The key determinants of health within Inuit communities identified in the ITK report include quality of early childhood development, culture and language, livelihoods, income distribution, housing, personal safety and security, education, food security, availability of health services, mental wellness, and the environment.

It is worth noting that these social determinants of health are considered in light of challenges, as well as identifying key positive efforts in each of these areas. For example, progressive efforts include learning and understanding constructs such as harm reduction, leadership development in communities, promoting Inuit language and culture, food security, and promoting culturally relevant services that focus on mental health and community well-being to address concerns about suicide. There are deep concerns about suicide among youth and young adults, and efforts at prevention are important to each community. Suicide is considered a serious health issue that contributes to chronic grief and loss. *Social Determinants of Inuit Health in Canada* (ITK 2014) is a critical and progressive report that is focused on health promotion. This report also highlights the work of the Maternal Child Health Working Group, which is working on supporting and promoting "healthy pregnancy and birthing by bringing birthing closer to home and preventing children being born with FASD" (13). It is also recognized that Inuit culture was disrupted through Canada's residential school experience in the Northwest Territories, which we address in relation to its relevance in this chapter.

Contextualizing the Topic of FASD in Northern Communities

Residential schools are part of the history of the North, and when children were moved far away from home, "many Inuit children lost their familial, communal, and socio-cultural connections, had no opportunity to eat country foods, were banned from speaking Inuit languages, and were forced to follow southern norms" (ITK 2007, 6). The removal of children from their communities to attend residential school has also left a legacy that resulted in broken ties in families due to this imposed separation. The legacy of these experiences contributes to the use of alcohol in communities in the Northwest Territories, and the intergenerational effects continue to unfold over time.

In reviewing the literature, the TRC—Virtual Quilt (Pauktuutit Inuit Women of Canada 2013) was discovered, which is a visual and artistic reflection based on the work of the Truth and Reconciliation Commission and the impact of residential schools in northern Canada. Similarly to our project, this project shares voices of women and men in communities who are reflecting on healing through the medium of artistic representations. The use of visual methodologies, then, reflects an important venue for sharing experience and voice.

It is very difficult to initiate and have conversations about FASD in small communities, given it is such a sensitive topic. Salmon and Clarren (2011) identified the need to develop culturally relevant responses to FASD prevention in the northern areas of Canada. It is critical to note that alcohol-exposed pregnancy is an experience grounded in historical trauma, and the use of alcohol is, more often than not, an effort to self-medicate against personal pain (Rutman 2011; Poole 2010). There is no intent to cause harm during pregnancy, yet judgmental viewpoints dominate in response to FASD. Prevention is not simply about abstention from alcohol during pregnancy, given that FASD is an outcome that is often a result of historical trauma. It is important to consider the interpersonal context for women that contributes to, and leads to, substance use. The identification of a child with FASD symbolically represents the need to look back at the history of the mother; prevention must be grounded in promoting health and healing for women, their families, and their communities. The health and healing journey is what makes a difference in prevention of many health and social challenges.

This project provided an opportunity to consider the topics of health and healing, while reflecting a positive approach to a dialogue through using visual imagery and text as a means to evoke reflection. Embarking on new pathways and having new conversations have a ripple effect in communities, which is resonant with Inuit societal values (Government of Nunavut 2013).

Approach to the Research

Given the challenges associated with the topic of FASD prevention, it was important to identify an approach to the topic that would contribute to a deeper understanding of the phenomenon of women's lived experience that deeply influences health choices over time. Photovoice was identified as the primary methodology for the Brightening Our Home Fires project as it is well suited to participatory action research (PAR).

Community members who live in, or have strong relational ties to, their communities were invited as co-researchers in this project. The research team held many discussions about how best to approach this topic, and over time it became clear that a focus on health and healing was an essential place to begin our exploration. It was also important to be transparent and identify that, while FASD is a health/social concern, the underlying construct of women's experience and health are contributing factors that require a much deeper understanding. Through the visual methodology of Photovoice and a qualitative research approach, women were asked to take photos in their home communities in response to the question: What does health and healing look like for you in your community?

Methodology

Photovoice was used as a primary methodology in this project, and it supports community engagement and involvement. PAR has created protocols for ensuring respectful and ethical partnerships that better support active and collaborative community participation in research (Aurora Research Institute [ARI] 2010). Photovoice as a methodology has traditionally focused on how a group of participants view a particular topic within their community (Palibroda et al. 2009). However, it was important to adapt Photovoice to work with individuals, as the topic is sensitive. Our adaptation involved working with individual women throughout the project.

Ethics Statement

Specific protocols exist for obtaining ethics for research in the Northwest Territories. This included completing an application for the Aurora Research Institute, NT, for a research licence, which takes several months to finalize and receive approval for. The waiting period is associated with the process of the ARI reviewing the application and engaging in community consultation in all communities where the research is to take place. It is also important to obtain letters of support to include in the application to ARI from communities where research will be conducted. Simultaneously, ethics approval for this project was obtained through the University of Calgary Conjoint Faculties Research Ethics Board. Once the university ethics certificate was obtained, the certificate was forwarded to ARI, at which point final approval was gained and a research licence granted. These measures are critical steps in the interest of transparency regarding research projects conducted in the Northwest Territories. While this process is detailed and lengthy, it is an essential aspect of conducting research that is respectful of northern communities in Canada.

Photovoice Examples and Reflection

In order to illustrate the representations of community and culture brought forth through Photovoice, co-author Annie Goose has shared several of her images and text created in this project. We also provide some images and text that women graciously shared in the project to give a sense of the process and content of the Photovoice project and the diverse images that represented health and well-being to the participants. Annie acted as host and translator, and also participated in the project. The northern reality is that all community members are welcome when a project takes place, and we are deeply appreciative of the involvement and voices of women that have contributed to a deeper understanding of health and healing grounded in community. Please note that all images and descriptive text for each photo in this chapter are used with consent.

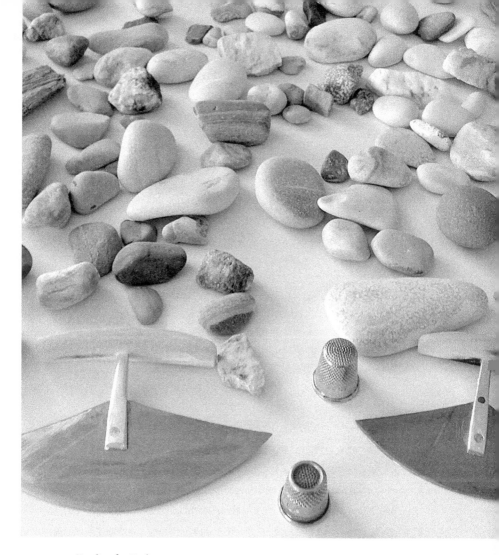

FIGURE 9.2 *Handicraft—Rocks.*

Handicraft—Rocks

My mom's handicraft of clothing she made was appreciated by us and that
is where I learned to do my best for my family and myself. She was a hard
worker and displayed her faith by doing rather than by talking. In my own
work and healing, I model what I have learned throughout my life—to share
with care, with those around me, my family, my community and anyone else.

— PHOTO BY ANNIE GOOSE, Ulukhaktok, NT, 2012

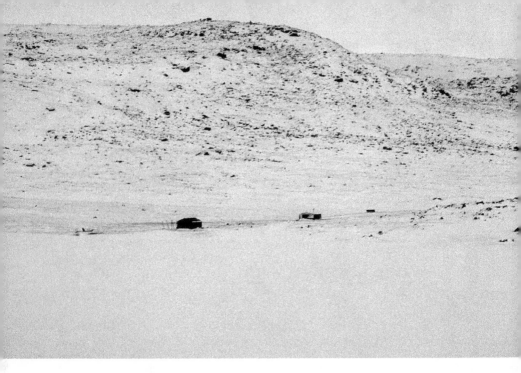

FIGURE 9.3 *The Land.*

The Land

The land—is my place of therapy, picturesque scenery, flowers, the stones, the rocks, the plants, animals, birds, ocean mammals all have a place in my own life. There was a time in my own life that I did not know how to properly prepare these things as a young mother, and over time I learned these skills, and how to store away dry, frozen meat and the lands has a way for my own life. I feel free, energy—you can gather energy wide as your arms, high as the sky and as deep as the ocean for your own life. If I am in the tree-line country I improvise—take in what I can and leave the rest.

— PHOTO BY ANNIE GOOSE, Ulukhaktok, NT, 2012

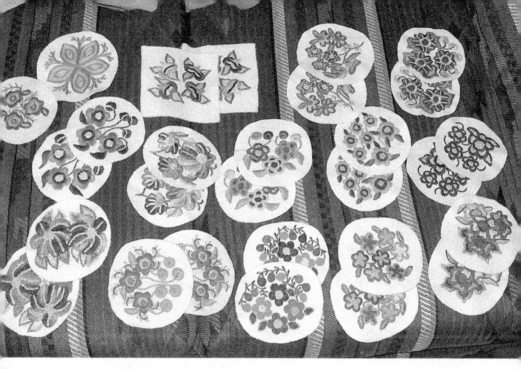

FIGURE 9.4 *My Work*.

My Work

Part of my therapy is through my handicrafts, which is very relaxing in creating
the colours and the choice of colours—the colours I choose reflect my healing
and how far I have come. I have a need to see the mistakes I make sometimes in my own life and reflect on how beautiful life, on my own, life can be
through my creations...As I do my handicrafts it helps me to relax and take
pride in my work and be real in my own healing journey. As I grow older and
progress in life I begin to know my own need to model and not so much speak
it or show it off. I need to be real in my own choices because life is about
choices and I know if I do make my choices I will live with either the positive
or the negative.

— PHOTO BY ANNIE GOOSE, Ulukhaktok, 2012

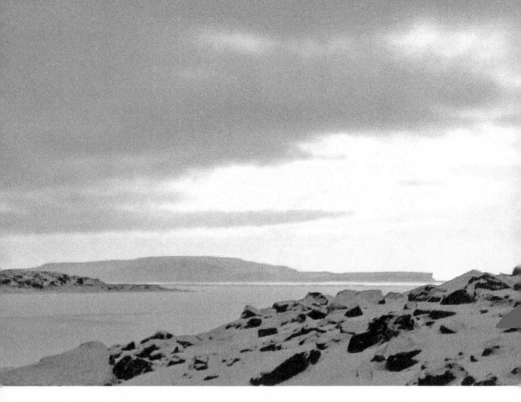

FIGURE 9.5 *A Light at the End of the Tunnel.*

A Light at the End of the Tunnel

This picture represents our greater power—the amazing gifts He has for people. No matter how dark things may seem there's always "a light at the end of the tunnel." There is always hope for a better tomorrow.

— PHOTO BY LAVERNA KLENGENBERG, Ulukhaktok, 2012

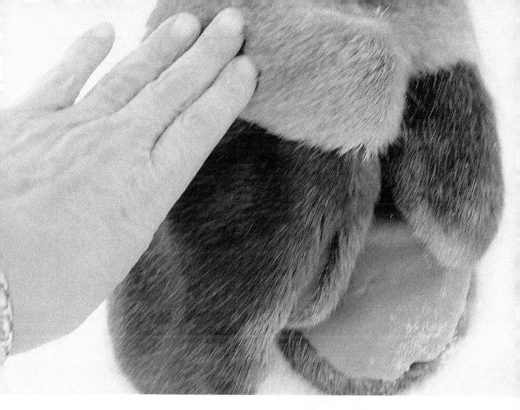

FIGURE 9.6 *Healing with Art.*

Healing with Art Photo

My crafts helped me to heal during a difficult part of my life. They help me express what I feel—they help me to think in quietness and contemplate life. My crafts are an expression of my thoughts, my dreams, and my hope for a better life. It is in these moments of sewing, of feeling, of thinking, of dreaming, of hoping, that I am who I can become. I am me, the way I really see myself.

— PHOTO BY LAVERNA KLENGENBERG, Ulukhaktok, 2012

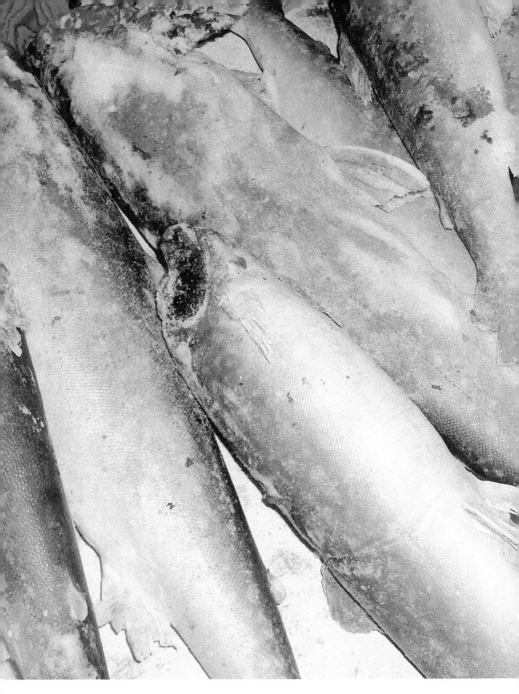

FIGURE 9.7 *Our Land—Our Country Food.*

UPLAK KOVIANATOK. KAOMANIK TAKOPLOGO. HILA.
PINIKTOK NONAMI MANIKKAMI NIGYOTIN. TAKOPLOGIN.
HAIMAKTIGOTAOKMATA NIKKIGHAK. KAITAOHIMAYOK NONAMON.
INOYUTTIKHAK KOYAGAMA. KOLVEK. KOVEMAN. NAMAATKA.
OKILIYOTTUN. ILIMATA.KOVIANAKNIK. MALILAGO. TAVONGA.
MAKITKIKPALUNGA. KANOLUNIN. MAMAKMA. DATIMALU
ILIHAOYUTAIT. ELANI. TAKOPLUGIN. MIGHONIK. MINGOLIHINIK.
ATOHUGO. TOGHIANIK ATOHUGO KUVIAKON. KAGLILIPAKTOK.
HILA. TAKOPLUGO.

Our Land, Our Country Food
Beautiful morning, bright and welcoming here in our community and our
region. Healing comes in many ways, through our culture and country food
chain, gives me strength for my physical and mental/emotional well-being,
through my tears that flow freely, gives me inner peace and healing. My
mother and father's words of encouragement, and through my artwork/crafts,
also my faith all are entwined together. Gives me my complete together as in
my recovery and my inner healing throughout life.[1]
— PHOTO BY ELSIE KLENGENBERG, Ulukhaktok, 2012

In summary, it is clear through all the beautiful photographs and captions
associated with each image that meaning is found in the everyday things
of life. It is important in community-based research to watch it unfold over
time. As co-authors, Annie and I have continued to collaborate since this
project ended and have participated together in conference presentations in
Edmonton, AB, and in Yellowknife, NT, at the first FASD conference in 2014.
We have also worked on several research articles and reports related to the
Brightening Our Home Fires project. As we worked through this chapter, and
talked about how we could present the research, we engaged in a reflective
conversation in the fall of 2015—three years after the project concluded. While
Annie spoke, I diligently typed each word.

Annie Goose Reflects on the Brightening Our Home Fires Project

One of the greatest most helpful ways of healing was captured in every person that participated in this project. In terms of healing personal family circle and always hoping our own version of recovery through PV was helpful to other people who are interested in this work. We know that personal wellness only happens when an individual comes to a place of needing to start enjoying life in general. Despite whatever challenges, setbacks, and times of feeling: Where do I go from here? And always looking up and getting back on board to continue healing, to enjoy life no matter what is about us in our daily lives.

And to forever continue role modelling, even though I may not always feel I am modelling my healing—even though recovery is about that. The impact of this project on the community is to see individual participants feel lightened—that Photovoice work was something to brighten individual living day to day. Through picture and words of encouragement, coming together was a very nonthreatening way of expressing—for where one was in their journey and where they want to go. Photovoice is real—the photos and one's words are real powerful. The focus on health and healing was also nonthreatening, and women felt free to express themselves through the question that was asked about health and healing.

Even though that project ended, the desire to do more Photovoice work exists. I think from the time that we started to work on something that looks at what type of need exists in personal healing. What kind of work can we do together in communities that is inviting to an individual who might want to participate—who might want to be part of a project that promotes self-healing? Photovoice has a large role for communities, particularly remote communities, and it's needed to open dialogue with people who feel they might be stuck in something and have no way to express those feelings and thoughts. How can I move on? What can I do? And to have trust built to express self, to feel included, and from that to continue moving forward. I feel there is a lot of room in any community to have Photovoice or other types of projects to happen in their community, to feel supported and to be asked if they would like to participate and carry on from there. Funding is always a need in the community for promoting healing and wellness in families. Photovoice has done a great deal for me as an individual! It's brought me forward to enjoy life, enjoy community, connections, and to understand when one is in the place of unsureness or uncertainties, and to do a project that is fun to do. There was enjoyment in taking photos and comparing that with person, emotion, mental space—it is a very safe way of expressing, and at the same time coming together with something that is very useful, colourful, strengthening ways for physical, emotional, mental. In hoping that it may help others to participate—there is always room, but it needs coordinators and people to take on projects, and for funders to work with communities to be open to work with communities in dialogue and to support other projects in the future.

The Findings: Key Themes Important to Health and Healing

In this section, the cumulative findings of the Brightening Our Home Fires project that involved four communities in the Northwest Territories is reflected. All the images and texts were entered into a qualitative software program called ATLAS.ti, then coded and analyzed for emerging themes. These themes were repeatedly identified in relation to health and healing and reflect the voices of women participants in response to the question: What does health and healing look like for you in your community? The themes are presented in alphabetical order below and are relevant to culture, place, and community health and healing.

- *Arts, Crafts, and Handiwork*: Women shared the cultural connection as reflected in these activities and found this work to be soothing and healing.
- *Community Care and Support*: Women reflected on the importance of being part of a community and being supported where they are at in life.
- *Employment (Work and Education)*: Women reflected that these were important factors, particularly in relation to the high cost of living in the Northwest Territories. Additionally, work opportunities were highlighted as severely limited in the Northwest Territories, and this presented both social and economic challenges.

- *Environment and the Land; Family (Children and Relatives)*: The environment is an integrated landscape that includes the land and family members (children, grandchildren, and extended family and relations). The importance of Elders was also highlighted in this theme, and their voices are deeply meaningful to the women. Elders also represent cultural connectedness through language preservation.

- *Health and Healing (Addiction)*: Almost all the women involved in this project had experiences with addiction, treatment, and recovery. There were many voices that reflected losses associated with addictions. Some women reflected that perhaps life could have taken a different path—one that was less difficult. It was notable that women in Yellowknife who were homeless had multiple experiences of trauma. One woman had taken a photo of a clock, and when asked to describe this picture, she commented that she realizes she lost a lot of time in her life. Women typically saw themselves in a healing process while acknowledging that there is always a need to stay connected to recovery resources, such as community members and counsellors who may provide telephone support in remote locations. It was identified that women with addiction issues feel exposed to a great deal of harm, experience a lack of safety, and primarily are dealing with unresolved trauma. Women also raised concerns about accessing addictions treatment in a timely manner, particularly when located in remote and isolated communities. Women's voices also indicated that they require supports around pre-conception planning where addiction is a concern.

- *Housing and Poverty Reduction*: This theme reflects an ongoing challenge, as housing resources in the Northwest Territories are limited. The need for social housing that is affordable was highlighted, and even those with housing struggled with bills and the high cost of living. Women participants who experienced homelessness in Yellowknife were particularly challenged, and many had lived in the shelter system for years.

- *Photovoice Project Participation and Connection with Culture*: Women identified that participating in this project gave them something to do, and it helped individuals to reflect on culture, as this was often the focus of photographs. One woman commented on her friends being mad at her for not hanging out with them while she participated in the project. One woman thought she might sell her camera, and she was asked to consider holding off for a couple of days. With great enthusiasm, this woman returned with twenty-seven photographs for which she provided deep reflections. One woman who agreed to participate eventually shared that she had given her camera to her son for his birthday, as she didn't have anything else to give him. Women were excited about receiving a camera to keep and taking a workshop on digital photography, as well as taking photos and reflecting on this work in the context of the project.

· *Tradition, Culture, and Elders' Roles*: This was another important theme threaded throughout the photos and reflections by women. Many women took photos of Elders, if possible, and reflected on the importance of those relationships. Also many photos were taken of the land and nature. For example, one woman reflected on the importance of the tree to the earth, but also commented that the tree was very cold, and she knew what it was like to be outside in the cold.

The voices and participation of women from four different locations in the Northwest Territories offered these themes, and they were relevant themes to all participants. The one exception was the challenges faced by women in Yellowknife who experienced homelessness. While they valued and reflected these themes, there was a tangible sense of challenges they faced in keeping connections in an urban setting, and homelessness contributed to many other social and economic challenges. It was our experience that women who were located in their home communities were able to reflect and connect deeply to these themes.

Other themes identified included:

· *Mental Health*: Access and availability of mental health services for all communities in the North is critical based on resolving historical and intergenerational concerns while supporting healthy relationships.

· *Trauma*: Levels of trauma vary but exist consistently in many communities. Ongoing efforts to address trauma, whether historically based or current, are a foundation for individual, family, and community health.

- *Travel:* Travel is an essential service in the North to access health care services for women in rural and remote communities. Travel to urban centres, for medical treatment, tests, and other support services, is critical. The ability and resources to travel for health matters for women can be very stressful, and a key finding of this research is that travel should be considered as a social determinant of health in northern Canada.

Conclusion: FASD Prevention Is about Health and Healing

The foundation of health and healing are critical constructs in FASD prevention. Engaging in FASD prevention work in the North requires a culturally sensitive approach and a deep focus on the lives of women in community. Talking about FASD is a sensitive topic and one that needs to be carefully approached in the North. In many ways the identification of a research project focused on FASD prevention can pose a barrier to participation, and this work may be best housed within a maternal health context. Linking FASD prevention and addiction supports to other health-based initiatives in communities is helpful. It was recognized in this project that connections with communities were forged over time, through visits and presence. FASD prevention is grounded in supporting family and community health. It is important to note that the experience of homeless women is profoundly different from other communities, and these women spoke more frequently about troubles with addiction and loss of children to care.

As a qualitative methodology, Photovoice opens doors to dialogue in a nonthreatening way, and taking photos opens new ways for women to see their world. In the voice of one participant: "I never thought about healing through photography!" Asking about health and healing is holistic and inviting. Women participants shared deep insights, and evoking images focused on their lives and communities. Asking about FASD can be a barrier in prevention activities. Photovoice supports developing and sharing new knowledge. Through this research, we were able to connect with women who were willing to share insights into their lives through Photovoice. We know that women are the best teachers about their health and healing processes, as well as shared aspects of community life including nature, culture, and the value of relationships. A camera is a tool that can effectively be used to engage in dialogues about complex health topics.

Acknowledgements

We acknowledge and truly thank all of the thirty women who were willing to share of themselves and offer insights into their lives through the Brightening Our Home Fires project. A special thanks goes to Laverna Klengenberg and Elsie Klengenberg for their contributions to this chapter. We would also like to thank the following:

- The First Nations and Inuit Health Branch for funding the project.
- The leadership and membership of the communities of Yellowknife, Łutselk'e, Behchokǫ̀, and Ulukhaktok for letters of support, community consultation, and engagement with the project.
- The Aurora Research Institute for consultation and granting a licence, and Dr. Pertice Moffitt, Yellowknife, NT, for her ongoing support and consultation on the project.
- The University of Calgary Conjoint Faculties Research Ethics Board for ethics review.
- All members of the research team, including members of the Canada FASD Research Network Action Team on Women's Health, Dorothy Badry, Dr. Amy Salmon, Arlene Hache, Marilyn Van Bibber, Dr. Aileen Wight Felske, Sandra Lockhart, and Dr. Nancy Poole, lead of the NAT on Women's Health/FASD Prevention.
- Dr. Christine Walsh from the University of Calgary, and Yellowknife photographer Tessa MacIntosh for acting as Photovoice consultants.
- The Canada FASD Research Network.

NOTE

1.   Translated from Kangiryuarmiutun by Annie Goose.

REFERENCES

Ajunnginiq Centre, National Aboriginal Health Organization. 2006. *Fetal Alcohol*
    Spectrum Disorder: An Environmental Scan of Services and Gaps in Inuit
    Communities. http://www.naho.ca/documents/it/2006_Inuit_FASD_scan.pdf.

Aurora Research Institute (ARI). About Licensing Research. https://nwtresearch.com/
    licensing.

Cameron, E. 2011. *State of the Knowledge: Inuit Public Health 2011.* National Collaborating
    Centre for Aboriginal Health. http://nccah.netedit.info/docs/setting%20the%20
    context/1739_InuitPubHealth_EN_web.pdf.

Canada FASD Research Network Action Team on Women's Health. 2010. *10 Fundamental*
    Components of FASD Prevention from a Women's Health Determinants Perspective.
    Vancouver: Canada Northwest FASD Research Network. http://www.canfasd.ca/files/
    PDF/ConsensusStatement.pdf.

Government of the Northwest Territories. 2014–2015. *Annual Report of the Director of*
    Child and Family Services 2014–2015, Including the Years 2006–2007 to 2014–2015.
    http://www.assembly.gov.nt.ca/sites/default/files/td_352-175.pdf.

Government of the Northwest Territories. 2015–2016. *Annual Report of the Director of*
    Child and Family Services 2015–2016, Including the Years 2006–2007 to 2015–2016.
    http://www.hss.gov.nt.ca/sites/hss/files/resources/cfs-directors-report-2015-2016.pdf.

Government of the Northwest Territories. 2019. *Mind and Spirit: Promoting Mental*
    Health and Addictions Recovery in the Northwest Territories. Mental Wellness
    and Addictions Recovery Action Plan. https://www.hss.gov.nt.ca/en/content/
    mental-wellness-and-addictions-recovery-action-plan.

Government of Nunavut. 2013. *Incorporating Inuit Societal Values.* http://www.ch.gov.
    nu.ca/en/Incorporating%20Inuit%20Societal%20Values%20Report.pdf.

Inuit Tapiriit Kanatami (ITK). 2007. *Social Determinants of Inuit Health in Canada.*
    http://ahrnets.ca/files/2011/02/ITK_Social_Determinants_paper_2007.pdf.

Inuit Tapiriit Kanatami (ITK). 2014. *Social Determinants of*
    Inuit Health in Canada. https://www.itk.ca/publication/
    comprehensive-report-social-determinants-inuit-health-national-inuit-organization.

Northwest Territories Health and Social Services. 2014. *Building Stronger Families: An*
    Action Plan to Transform Child and Family Services. https://www.hss.gov.nt.ca/en/
    resources?f%5B0%5D=field_resource_category%3A169&page=1.

Northwest Territories Health and Social Services. 2011. *Health Status Report.* http://www. hlthss.gov.nt.ca/pdf/reports/health_care_system/2011/english/nwt_health_status_ report.pdf.

Northwest Territories Health and Social Services. 2015. *Report on Substance Use and Addiction.* March 2015. http://www.hss.gov.nt.ca/sites/hss/files/report-on-substance-use-and-addiction-2012.pdf.

Palibroda, B., B. Krieg, L. Murdock, and J. Havelock. 2009. *A Practical Guide to Photovoice: Sharing Pictures, Telling Stories and Changing Communities.* Winnipeg: The Prairie Women's Health Centre of Excellence. http://www.pwhce.ca/photovoice/pdf/ Photovoice_Manual.pdf.

Pauktuutit Inuit Women of Canada. 2010. *Inuit Five-Year Plan for Fetal Alcohol Spectrum Disorder: 2010–2015.* Ottawa: Pauktuutit Inuit Women of Canada Press.

Pauktuutit Inuit Women of Canada. 2013. TRC—Virtual Quilt. Nipiqaqtugut Sanaugatigut. https://pauktuutit.ca/abuse-prevention-justice/residential-schools/ trc-virtual-quilt-nipiqaqtugut-sanaugatigut/.

Poole, N. 2010. "Bringing a Women's Health Perspective to FASD Prevention." In *Fetal Alcohol Spectrum Disorder: Management and Policy Perspectives of FASD,* edited by E. Riley, S. Clarren, J. Weinberg, and E. Jonsson, 161–74. Hoboken, New Jersey: Wiley-Blackwell.

Rutman, D. 2011. *Substance Using Women with FASD and FASD Prevention. Voices of Women with FASD: Promising Approaches in Substance Use Treatment and Care.* Victoria: University of Victoria.

Salmon, A., and S.K. Clarren. 2011. "Developing Effective, Culturally Appropriate Avenues to FASD Diagnosis and Prevention in Northern Canada." *International Journal of Circumpolar Health* 70, no. 4 (September): 428–33. https://pubmed.ncbi.nlm.nih. gov/21878184/.

Wang C., and M.A. Burris. 1997. "Photovoice: Concept, Methodology, and Use for Participatory Needs Assessment." *Health Education & Behavior* 24, no. 3: 369–87. doi:10.1177/109019819702400309.

World Health Organization. 2008. *Closing the Gap in a Generation: Health Equity through Action on the Social Determinants of Health.* Final Report of the Commission on Social Determinants of Health. https://apps.who.int/iris/bitstream/handle/10665/43943/9789 241563703_eng.pdf.

World Health Organization. 2013. *Social Determinants of Health.* http://www.who.int/ social_determinants/en/.

10 Traditional Knowledge, Science, and Protection

MARC FONDA

Marc Fonda was an adjunct research professor in sociology at the University of Western Ontario at the time of writing this chapter, and had a long career in policy research at the Social Science and Humanities Research Council of Canada and at what is now Indigenous Services Canada. He has a long-standing interest in issues of Traditional Knowledge of Indigenous Peoples, and in issues of Indigenous intellectual property and its protection. This chapter is based on a presentation he gave at the Wisdom Engaged: Traditional Knowledge for Northern Community Well-Being conference, which took place in Edmonton, Alberta, in February 2015.[1]

Introduction

Traditional Knowledge of Indigenous and local peoples the world over is increasingly recognized as valuable and salient. The World Intellectual Property Organization (n.d.) defines *Traditional Knowledge* as "knowledge, know-how, skills and practices that are developed, sustained and passed on from generation to generation within a community, often forming part of its cultural or spiritual identity." It further reminds us that "Traditional knowledge can be found in a wide variety of contexts, including: agricultural, scientific, technical, ecological and medicinal knowledge as well as biodiversity-related knowledge." Traditional Knowledge thus provides insight into aspects of human and animal/plant nature, local environments, resources, and world views. Fikret Berkes has provided the most widely cited definition of traditional ecological knowledge, which is "a cumulative body of knowledge, practice and belief evolving by adaptive processes and handed down through generations by cultural transmission, about the relationship of living beings (including humans) with one another and with their environment" (1999, 8). As a knowledge-practice belief complex, traditional ecological knowledge includes the world view or religious traditions of a society. "It is both cumulative and dynamic, building on experience and adapting to changes" (Berkes 1999, 8), as societies constantly redefine what is considered "traditional." Further, Felice Wyndham reminds us that the living relations of knowing and acting, and the "phenomenological experience of traditional ecological knowing is inescapably relational and transactional, best characterized by the way it activates or mediates interaction" (2017, 78). In this chapter, the relationship with nature is implied when the term *Traditional Knowledge* is used.

The value of Traditional Knowledge has been recognized by institutions like the United Nations (UN) and the World Health Organization (WHO). The UN's Declaration on the Rights of Indigenous Peoples (UN 2008), for instance, recognizes that "respect for indigenous knowledge, cultures and traditional practices contributes to sustainable and equitable development and proper management of the environment" (2). In fact, Article 11.1 "includes the right to maintain, protect and develop the past, present and future manifestations of their cultures, such as archaeological and historical sites, artefacts, designs, ceremonies, technologies and visual and performing arts and literature." And Article 11.2 declares, "States shall provide redress through effective mechanisms, which may include restitution, developed in conjunction with indigenous peoples, with respect to their cultural, intellectual, religious and spiritual property taken without their free, prior and informed consent or in violation of their laws, traditions and customs" (6).

The UN Declaration of the Rights of Indigenous Peoples recognizes de facto the value of traditional Indigenous knowledge and requires signatory states to provide redress where necessary.

The World Health Organization also values Traditional Knowledge, and for good reason. Its 2002–2005 and 2014–2023 Traditional Medicine Strategies outline the value of Traditional Knowledge in relation to health care. Both underline the importance of Traditional Knowledge in providing health care services, in particular in countries that lack a comprehensive health care system (WHO 2002, 2013, 28). For instance, in many African countries the ratio of Traditional Healers to the population is 1:500, whereas the ratio of medical doctors to the population is 1:40,000 (27). Clearly, traditional medicine is a viable option, providing front-line health care to a large number of people. The WHO Traditional Medicine Strategies also recognize the increasing use of complementary and alternative medicines[2] in countries with comprehensive health care systems. In fact, the 2014–2023 version notes that, in 2011, 70 per cent of Canadians used complementary and alternative medicines, and that the global market for herbal medicines in 2003 was over $60 billion USD annually and growing steadily (WHO 2003).

The purpose of this chapter is to review and explore various aspects of Traditional Knowledge as it relates to its importance, the differences between Traditional Knowledge and scientific knowledge, and some of the challenges that intellectual property regimes bring to preserving and protecting Traditional Knowledges. I also look at some international initiatives to provide such protection that can act as models for improvement. In doing this, I offer an overview of the role that traditional Indigenous and local knowledges play and can continue to play in contemporary societies.

The Importance of Traditional Knowledge

The literature on Traditional Knowledge is wide-ranging and expanding. Much of this literature historically has not been written by Indigenous people (Simpson 1999, 2001), and it has been concerned with how Traditional Knowledge relates to a variety of issues such as natural resource extraction and biocultural diversity, climate change, knowledge transmission and preservation, and the well-being of and benefits to the people from which the Traditional Knowledge comes, and tensions between these issues.

During the colonial period, exploitation of traditional Indigenous knowledge led to wealth through resource exploitation and commercialization of Indigenous medicines and foods (see Balick and Cox [2021] for a discussion of the history of herbal medicines during the colonial period). More recently, interest in Traditional Knowledge has expanded into other markets, such as the pharmaceutical industry, seed industry, agro forestry, and the New Age book market. The exploitation of Traditional Knowledge has yielded substantial funds, but the beneficiaries of this enterprise have rarely been Indigenous or local peoples. In 1990, ethnobiologist Darrell Posey estimated that the profits related to medicines derived from medicinal plants originally discovered by Indigenous Peoples were around $43 billion USD, while at the same time there was a $25 billion USD seed industry. Yet, in 1989, less than 0.001 per cent of these profits were returned to Indigenous Peoples the world over. More recently, the United Nations University (2012) reported estimates that the worldwide annual market value for herbal medicines alone was around $60 billion USD. Since then, in 2019, the WHO estimated the global herbal medicine market to be $83 billion USD, and it expects it to exceed $411 billion USD by 2026 (WHO 2019). It would seem that biological resources are a form of capital with vast economic potential—especially in places with intact landscapes. As Aguilar (2001) noted some time ago, biodiversity is important not only to the natural sciences but also in economic and social spheres.

Traditional Knowledge is also important to economic equity. During the 1950s and 1960s, Traditional Knowledge was seen as inefficient, inferior, and an obstacle to development intended to transform societies in the model of Euro-North American industrial economies. This changed gradually as people increasingly recognized the importance of Traditional Knowledge to agricultural production systems and sustainable development (Agrawal 1995). By the 1970s, development practitioners started to see Traditional Knowledge as an essential element to success (Agrawal 1995; Aguilar 2001). For Agrawal (1995), the concept of Traditional Knowledge was reified by development practitioners and theorists alike. It has since been viewed as the latest and best strategy to fight hunger, poverty, social inequity, and environmental racism. It has been especially pivotal in discussions of sustainable resource use and climate change. Legal scholar Anthony Moffa (2016), however, notes that, despite the recognition of the importance of Traditional Knowledge in numerous scientific and technical fields, there has been very little use of it as a substantive basis for administrative policy making in the United States (outside of Alaska), Canada, and globally.

There has been a great deal written on the protection of Traditional Knowledge since the 1990s, in response to the recognition of the value of Traditional Knowledge with concerns about preserving biocultural diversity (Maffi and Woodley 2010; North America Regional Declaration on Biocultural Diversity 2019), and to the growing conception of Indigenous intellectual property as central to identity and sovereignty. Many Indigenous Peoples have had their knowledge and heritage taken from them with no or minimal compensation, and their relationship to and rights to their traditional territories ignored by the nation-states in which their homelands are located (Simpson 2001). Indeed, concerns regarding protection are based on fundamental justice issues; that is, the right to expect a fair return on, and the right to use and protect, that which communities have invented or developed (Government of Canada n.d.; Mugabe 1999). Simply said, as the awareness of Traditional Knowledge grows in mainstream society, so does the risk of its misappropriation in the form of image rights, use of plants without compensation, and selling philosophical insights by non-Indigenous spiritual entrepreneurs. Non-Indigenous people ought to recognize a motivation to ensure the fair use of Traditional Knowledge, since it has much to offer contemporary societies. In Canada, Traditional Knowledge is increasingly used to inform policy making related to food and agriculture, culture, human rights, resource management, sustainable development, and the conservation of biological diversity, health, trade, and economic development (Government of Canada n.d.).

Finally, Traditional Knowledge is central to the well-being of Indigenous communities and peoples. Castellano (2009) notes that Traditional Knowledge helps bridge the historical distance between Indigenous Peoples and settler cultures, as it defies assimilation myths and pressure from the dominance of Western scientific knowledge. In speaking about Inuit in Canada, Tulloch (2009) indicates that the Inuit language promotes bridging and social bonding by bringing generations closer together, sharing Traditional Knowledge and skills, and that finding one's place in the world provides cultural agency. Chandler and Lalonde's (2008) important work on suicide in British Columbia's First Nations communities demonstrates that the greater the "cultural continuity" within a community, the lower the suicide rates. Their work focuses on the importance of self-determination and agency at both the individual and community levels. They found that individual and cultural continuity are closely linked, and that those communities that have success in preserving their cultural heritage and ensuring their sovereignty are significantly better at insulating their youth from suicide. The current level of interest in Traditional Knowledge is about improving the well-being of Indigenous Peoples, whether it is in the form of increasing food and medicine security, promoting well-being, intergenerational knowledge exchange, or profit sharing.

Differences between Traditional Knowledge and Scientific Knowledge

Mississauga Nishnaabeg scholar Leanne Betasamosake Simpson (2001) points out that many Indigenous people may take issue with the fact the term *Traditional Knowledge* was "largely defined and developed as a concept outside of Aboriginal communities" (139), and have problems with the way it is defined, which reflects what the dominant societies see as important. She also notes the irony that Traditional Knowledge is now being sought as a solution to the environmental degradation that colonialism has caused (2004). Like Anishanaabe scholar Deborah McGregor (2008), from the viewpoint of natural and environmental justice, Simpson (2001) and Mohawk scholar Mary Arquette et al. (2002) state that the communities most affected have a right to be at the table, fully using their knowledge in culturally safe environments to make decisions impacting their communities and peoples. While some scholars argue that holistic Indigenous knowledge and ways of environmental planning surpass the reductionist approach of Western societies (LaDuke 1994; Simpson 2001; McGregor 2008; Moffa 2016), others claim that Traditional Knowledge is not as effective as sciencitifc knowledge. Such claims are often based on substantive, methodological and epistemological, and contextual grounds. Substantively, there are differences in the subject matter and characteristics of the two knowledge systems. In terms of methodology and epistemology, differences arise from varying investigative methods. Contextual differences stem from Traditional Knowledge being deeply rooted in the local environment and its social and spiritual context, whereas scientific knowledge is not (Agrawal 1993; Berkes 1999; Simpson 2001; Kimmerer 2002; McGregor 2008).

Despite such claims, Arun Agrawal (1993) argues that there is no sustainable difference between Traditional Knowledge and scientific knowledge. He notes that much of this kind of thinking is rooted in early anthropology's dichotomy of "primitive" and "modern" societies. For instance, Agrawal describes how Levi-Strauss (1967) suggested that primitive cultures are more embedded in their environments than modern cultures; are less prone than scientific investigators to use analytic reasoning that might question the foundations of that knowledge; and, Traditional Knowledge systems are more closed than science knowledge systems. This is a form of reification of Traditional Knowledge, which has led to difficulties by dichotomizing knowledge and attempting to reclassify, abstract, and generalize Traditional Knowledge for scientific knowledge purposes (Agrawal 1993).

Are there substantive differences between Traditional Knowledge and scientific knowledge? Agrawal (1993) points out that there is a presumption that Traditional Knowledge is concerned with immediate and concrete necessities of people's daily livelihoods, and that scientific knowledge attempts to generate general explanations that are abstracted from daily lives. This view is not sustainable. There is scarcely any part of modern life that does not bear the imprint of science. While there are differences between philosophies and several forms of knowledge commonly viewed as Traditional Knowledge or scientific knowledge, there are also approaches separated by this divide that share substantial similarities, such as agro forestry, tree-cropping systems, taxonomy, and plant classifications. Moreover, this classification of Traditional Knowledge and scientific knowledge fails on a more fundamental level: it seeks to separate and fix in time and space knowledge systems that can never be so separated or fixed (see also McGregor 2008).

Are there methodological or epistemological differences between Traditional Knowledge and scientific knowledge? Some researchers claim that scientific knowledge is open, systematic, objective, analytic, and advances by building rigorously on prior achievements, whereas Traditional Knowledge is seen as closed, nonsystemic, holistic rather than analytic, and advances on the basis of new experiences not deductive logic (Agrawal 1993; McGregor 2008). This distinction recalls the failure of many philosophers of science (e.g., Leibniz, Popper) to find satisfactory lines of demarcation between science and nonscience. Most have long abandoned the hope of a satisfactory method of doing so. For instance, as Agrawal (1993) continues, Feyerabend's (1975) attacks on scientific dogmatism and intolerance of insights gained outside institutional science were good enough that his avowed critics accepted them. Two decades later, Dirks, Eley, and Ortner (1994) noted it was the virtual absence of historical investigations in anthropology that made cultural systems appear timeless, at least until ruptured by contact. As such, it is impossible to insist on the openness of science when confronted by attempts aimed at dislodging it—a perspective also supported by Kuhn (1962)—or, for that matter, of the supposed closed nature of Traditional Knowledge systems.

Are there contextual differences between Traditional Knowledge and scientific knowledge? Traditional Knowledge is often seen as existing in local contexts, being anchored to a particular setting and time. In contrast, scientific knowledge is seen as divorced from local context and epistemic frameworks in the search for universal validity. Agrawal (1993) asks if such a distinction makes sense. He notes that one criticism levelled at developmental policies/programs is their ignorance of the social, political, and cultural contexts in which they are implemented. It is likely that development's so-called technical solutions are themselves as anchored in as specific a political, cultural, and temporal milieu as is Traditional Knowledge (Agrawal 1993). What this means is that science is fixed in a social context, and this fact brings into question its rationality and objectivity. It can be argued that science is a practice and a culture in and of itself; it is culturally bound and based on specific cultural interests (Franklin 1995). For this reason, it is very difficult to insist that scientific knowledge is not context-bound and does not respond to its own cultural demands any more than does Traditional Knowledge. There are different "recipes" for success in the literature. For example, Agrawal (1993) suggests that success will come from building new epistemic foundations, and that innovation and experimentation requires bridging Traditional Knowledge and scientific knowledge: "Instead of trying to conflate all non-Western knowledge into a category termed 'indigenous', and all Western knowledge into another category it may be more sensible to accept differences within these categories and perhaps find similarities across them" (5). Similarly, Tsuji and Ho (2002) see Traditional Knowledge's holistic approach as offering insight into complex, nonlinear systems in ways that scientific knowledge cannot, and encourage finding a way to integrate it more effectively.

Simpson (1999, 2001) and McGregor (2008) present a more nuanced appreciation of Traditional Knowledge, as it is embedded in culture through its physical, spiritual, and intellectual context. Indigenous Peoples are reluctant to allow scientists to interpret their knowledge as removed from the values and spiritual origins because, when this does happen, the knowledge is at risk of becoming an assimilated commodity that can be used at will by settler society to support existing doctrine and agendas. One needs to understand Traditional Knowledge as an epistemology that is rooted in the spiritual world and the language in which the knowledge is embedded, since "the knowledge can only be understood in reference of the world view" (Simpson 2001, 143).

For McGregor (2008), the terminology for *traditional ecological knowledge* is problematic: the phrase assumes a homogeneity to such knowledge across diverse nations and cultures. "Traditional" implies the knowledge is static and confined to the past; "ecological" limits Traditional Knowledge to a field of study defined by Western science; and the use of "knowledge" itself is problematic as Indigenous Peoples tend to describe traditional ecological knowledge as a way of life and should be seen more as a verb or process of relations than a noun or the possession of a thing. The solution is not isolation but a form of parallelism, described as following the Haudenosaunee model of the two-row wampum (McGregor 2008), where two sets of knowledge and ways of knowing are applied in parallel and equally to policy making according to their own world views. For Simpson and McGregor, it is not about the one type of knowledge assimilating or assuming the other, but a case of the two knowledge systems working in parallel to inform decision making.

Finally, from a legal studies viewpoint, McGonigle (2016) notes, "Taking indigenous worlds seriously necessitates recognizing that indigenous people may be living in different schemes of reality, or 'ontologies,' which can subsequently escape normative Western legal reasoning" (224). The solution to this challenge is recognizing ontological pluralism, which means taking seriously the narratives and visions "that sustain indigenous worlds, even if they conflict with normative assumptions and understandings" (225). McGonigle's point is that there is a need to take steps toward "symmetrical" exchanges that will bring the legal status of protection to Indigenous knowledges.

Challenges of Intellectual Property Regimes

Before the United Nations Declaration on the Rights of Indigenous Peoples (UN 2008), including the rights to free, prior, informed consent (FPIC), was available, the ownership and treatment of Traditional Knowledge lacked clear international and national rules. Adherence to FPIC has been slow globally, and so Indigenous and local peoples have seen uneven and often low control or financial benefits for outside access to their Traditional Knowledges. This underscores the role that states have in developing protections for biodiversity and creating the tools needed to define rights and obligations for different actors with regard to genetic and other resources found on the lands of Indigenous Peoples (see North American Regional Declaration on Biocultural Diversity 2019). As Aguilar (2001, 243) points out, "Clean and simple legislation that responds to the needs of each country is one of the key elements to ensure fair and equitable distribution of benefits." This approach ought to be informed actively by the participation of Traditional Knowledge holders as a sincere response to the concerns voiced by Indigenous participants in the debate over protecting intellectual property and data sovereignty (Simpson 1999, 2001; Arquette et al. 2002; McGregor 2008).

Ex situ preservation of Traditional Knowledge often takes the form of using databases to capture and render this information useful in other contexts.

According to Agrawal (2002), the use of databases to preserve Traditional Knowledge does not really work. For Agrawal (2002, 202, 291), "Statements that are successfully particularized, validated, and generalized become knowledge by satisfying a particular relationship between utility, truth, and power. The process of scientisation helps instantiate a division within indigenous knowledge systems so that only useful indigenous knowledge systems become worthy of protection." The logic of databases requires that Traditional Knowledge is "scientized," or transformed into something "useful," or assimilated by a dominant society (Simpson 2001). According to Agrawal (2002), this is done in a three-step process, where knowledge is particularized, validated, and generalized. These three steps can be seen as the basis of establishing truth content or a particular Traditional Knowledge-based practice. It can also "be seen as identical with truth-making," in that it helps Traditional Knowledge to emerge as a fact recognizable by scientific knowledge (Agrawal 2002).

1. *Particularizing Traditional Knowledge*: This step demands that Traditional Knowledge is separated from related knowledge and practices, its milieu and context, as the well as the cultural beliefs with which it exists in combination, because they are seen as irrelevant to the needs of "development" and can be allowed to pass away.

2. *Validating and Abstracting Traditional Knowledge*: This second step uses scientific criteria to homogenize information "elements" in a database. Here, particularized Traditional Knowledge is further abstracted to its essential core in the image of science (rejecting nonessential aspects) for it to be useful for development. Once validated, it can be included in a database.

3. *Generalizing Traditional Knowledge*: Once the Traditional Knowledge is abstracted and validated, it is archived, categorized, and circulated as "useful" knowledge, and only then can development activities start.

Despite the truth value of Indigenous knowledge systems, their perceived lack of utility renders them unsuitable for inclusion in development databases, which possess instrumental power in colonial policy initiatives. Being left out, those pieces of knowledge are deemed without any use and generally cannot be applied to advance claims in most cases. They become neither true nor false; they are simply unnecessary to those engaged in development and environmental conservation. And so, is there anything particularly Indigenous about knowledge that has undergone the sanitization implicit in scientization or being made database-ready? "In the very moment that indigenous knowledge is proved useful to development through the application of science, it is, ironically, stripped of the specific characteristics that could even potentially make it indigenous" (Agrawal 2002, 292; see also Simpson 2001; McGregor 2008). In this context, Traditional Knowledge is rendered into a form of scientific knowledge, rather than truly braiding the two systems.[3]

While scientized Traditional Knowledge often loses much of its cultural context, there have been times when databases have proven useful in Canada. For example, the Sciences Act (Sciences Act Administration 1988) requires that all scientific activities in Canada's territories (Yukon, Northwest, and Nunavut) obtain a licence from the territorial government. Researchers must disclose complete details on the research, its general goals, and maintenance of confidentiality, intellectual property arrangements, use of data, and how the information will be communicated back to the communities involved in the research. This act set a precedent in Canada and internationally, and helped to establish free, prior, and informed consent in the research process. More interestingly, the information in this database was used in land claim negotiations leading to the establishment of Nunavut. This suggests that databases for Traditional Knowledge can be used effectively (INAC/Government of Canada 1999). They can help establish practices that lead to solid and mutually beneficial contracts, which consider things like the period of the agreement, the terms of reference, the nature of community involvement, the ownership of intellectual property, what the different parties can do with Traditional Knowledge and intellectual property, as well as the amount, form, and method of compensation.

National intellectual property regimes generally offer protection to Traditional Knowledge in two ways. Some countries have enacted specific legislation establishing minimum standards for recognition and protection of Traditional Knowledge. In most jurisdictions, however, communities have made use of existing legal tools and intellectual property rights law to try to protect their Traditional Knowledge. They have had mixed success. Existing laws require that a product is original, innovative, or distinctive, and that it be disclosed before it can be acknowledged and protected. This approach favours corporations and innovation over communities and preservation. In fact, most national intellectual property regimes do not recognize communal ownership. (Two key but dated sources do open the discussion of community rights with regard to plants and traditional resource rights [see Posey and Dutfield 1996, and the Crucible Group 1994]). However, mechanisms to create this protection would require national legislation and reciprocal recognition in other countries, development of an international germplasm database, and some type of international ombudsman or public defender, according to the Crucible group. Moreover, Traditional Knowledge development takes place over long periods of time, therefore it is difficult to establish as distinct, innovative, or original.

In addition, costs associated with using intellectual property regimes can be prohibitive; the timing of such protections is limited (but can be renewed) and, with the exception of copyright protection, must be sought in many national jurisdictions; and coverage is spotty with little ability to enforce ownership (INAC/Government of Canada 1999). It seems that, "In Canada, effective domestic legislation that clearly protects Indigenous traditional knowledge has not yet been adopted. It falls directly on Indigenous communities, therefore, to ensure necessary measures are taken to protect their traditional knowledge" (Government of Canada n.d.). A more recent Government of Canada publication (2022) indicates intellectual property associated with innovations and artistic creations remains an area of challenge. It recognizes the difference in world views between settler society and Indigenous Peoples, and that current mechanisms are not adapted to these differences. It also notes that, in 2018, the Minister of Innovation, Science and Economic Development announced an intellectual property strategy and designed a web page for information on Indigenous Peoples and intellectual property.[4]

This is not to say that intellectual property tools are not available and are not being used by Indigenous Peoples. In Canada, there are multiple instances of Indigenous artists and musicians making use of copyright, and Indigenous-owned companies registering trademarks (e.g., OCAP®) and industrial designs (the West Baffin Eskimo Cooperative has fifty at least, for instance). Moreover, there are international initiatives that provide useful examples, including the Biodiversity Convention (UN 1992),[5] which established first principles for negotiation and relation of legal solutions at a national level, and acknowledges that Indigenous Peoples need to be included in initiatives, despite its weaknesses (as it asks but does not require states to follow the convention). The Biodiversity Convention (UN 1992) acknowledges the need for protection of Traditional Knowledge associated with genetic resources—such as the commercial use of genetic resources (articles 2, 15), and the commercial use of knowledge and innovations/practices of Indigenous and local communities (article 8j).

A second example is the International Labor Organization Convention 169 (1989) "Concerning Indigenous Peoples and Tribes in Independent Countries." This convention contains some important measures for protection of the rights of Indigenous Peoples and recognition of lands, territories, and use of resources. Part II, under the title "Lands," suggests an obligation to recognize the rights of Indigenous Peoples to property and to possess the lands that they have traditionally occupied, including the right to participate in the use, administration, and conservation of these resources. Other examples are the United Nations Declaration for the Rights of Indigenous People (UN 2008), Costa Rica's Biodiversity Law (Legislative Assembly of the Republic of Costa Rica 1998), the Third World Network's *Biodiversity, Traditional Knowledge and Rights of Indigenous Peoples* (Tauli-Corpuz 2004), the Universal Declaration of Rights of Mother Earth (World People's Conference on Climate Change and the Rights of Mother Earth 2010), India's *People's Biodiversity Register* (National Biodiversity Authority, India 2013), and the North American Regional Declaration on Biocultural Diversity (2019). Such existing international agreements and covenants and the Universal Declaration of Human Rights (UN 1948) provide hope but are all limited as legal instruments with respect to protecting Traditional Knowledge. In reference to intellectual property of ethnopharmaceutical knowledge, McGonigle (2016, 221) notes that international agreements "have not yet yielded the intended results of giving satisfactory 'scientific value' or protection of local resources, nor bring adequate benefits to indigenous communities." And a 2019 review of progress on the challenges Posey made in 1990 concludes that, while advances have been made, more needs to be done. Golan et al. (2019) suggest that progress has been incremental over the past decades, and there is a need for more international standards, given that the application of protocols are still left to national policy. Additionally, there is a lack of governing bodies nationally and internationally that deal with ethical issues related to Traditional Knowledge and intellectual property, and widespread use of vague language in international conventions or agreements often leads to legal ambiguity that leaves local communities vulnerable.

More initiatives have emerged since 2001. One striking example is the Biodiversity Act of Bhutan (Government of Bhutan 2003). This legislation applies a positive protection regime for plant varieties (Chapter 3), and directly addresses the rights afforded to Traditional Knowledge (Chapter 4). In this case, access to resources and Traditional Knowledge rights are tied to one another and includes guidelines for benefit sharing, in perpetuity, and inalienable rights to Traditional Knowledge. It provides the owner of Traditional Knowledge the right to reject application for rights to use resources or medicines gained from Traditional Knowledge.

Golan et al. (2019) discuss other examples. For instance, in 2005 South Africa passed an amended Patent Act, in which section 30:3B "requires that patent applicants provide proof of origin and specify the intended use of Indigenous or local biological resource" (Golan et al. 2019, 96), and South Africa has used section 30:3B successfully to protect such resources against a multinational corporation, Nestlé. Additionally, in 2004 Peru established national procedures to protect biological resources. Peru's National Commission Against Biopiracy was established and identified thirty-five biological resources, many which related to Traditional Knowledge, and has "campaigned successfully for the rejection, abandonment, or withdrawal of nine controversial patents" (Golan et al. 2019, 97). This is an impressive accomplishment, and can be a model for other countries, while there is still more need for the inclusion of Traditional Knowledge in policy making that ensures the well-being of Indigenous and local peoples.

I present here a brief review of some of the approaches suggested by key authors to ensure protection of and appropriate benefit from development of Traditional Knowledge. Various local and Indigenous groups have pursued many of these approaches over the past two decades, but it is worthwhile to briefly summarize them here. It appears that Agrawal is mainly speaking to international development professionals and researchers in much of his writing on this topic. He notes that innovation and experimentation requires bridging Traditional and scientific knowledges. "Instead of trying to conflate all non-Western knowledge into a category termed 'indigenous', and all Western knowledge into another category," Agrawal writes, "it may be more sensible to accept differences within these categories and perhaps find similarities across them" (1995, 5). Some Indigenous thinkers (i.e., Simpson 1999, 2001) and McGregor (2008) do not agree, continuing to find utility in recognition of Indigenous knowledge. Aguilar (2001), who writes mainly on genetic resources, suggests that national legislation ought to begin by recognizing the rights of Indigenous Peoples to sovereignty. This includes such customary rights as self-determination, property rights in land and natural resources, and the right to follow their own norms. He argues that national legislation is a critical tool for recognizing such rights. Issues of sovereignty between Indigenous Peoples and the nation-states in which their homelands are located complicate legislative approaches.

Conclusion

The bias of scientific knowledge over other forms of thinking is well established. This takes place in medical training and practice, as is visible in Western medicine's general disdain for alternate approaches to health care, despite the encouraging uptick of its use in Western societies. But, at the same time, an honest Western-trained doctor will tell you that most healing takes place in the mind, and they will emphasize that science does not yet well understand how the healing process works. As suggested earlier, those working from within the scientific paradigm are uncomfortable acknowledging or even assessing traditional practices related to alternate healing methods, and when they do, they use the categories of scientific and biomedical knowledge. This raises the question: Is such behaviour due to paradigmatic biases or fear of competition and loss of power?

It should be emphasized that the goal of Traditional Healing is not different from that of Western medicine. This alone ought to aid in breaking the barriers between Traditional Healing and "scientific" healing practices and cultures. However, there is the added challenge of addressing health inequities in places that lack well-established and comprehensive health care systems. This is the result not only of the erosion of Traditional Knowledge and related practices through the world, but it is also a result of the culture of medical education that further distances younger generations of traditional peoples from exploring Traditional Knowledge as related to healing.

There should be no doubt as to the value of Traditional Healing practices and medicines. As Alves and Rosa (2007) point out, 50 per cent of commercially available drugs are based on bioactive compounds extracted or patterned from nonhuman species. A great number of these natural products have come to us from the scientific study of remedies traditionally employed by various cultures. In other words, folk or traditional medicine uses "represent 'leads' that could shortcut the discovery of modern medicines" (Alves and Rosa 2007, 2). In addition, of the 119 known, useful, plant-derived drugs, "74% of the chemical compounds used as drugs have the same or related use as the plants from which they were derived" (Alves and Rosa 2007, 2). This alone should influence the protection and respect of Traditional Knowledges the world over.

Improvements have taken place. According to the WHO (2013), the number of member states that have a traditional medicine policy, and that regulate herbal medicines, has grown since 1999 from 25 and 65, to 69 and 119, respectively. The WHO also informs us that the number of countries with a traditional medicine strategy improved between 1999 and 2012, from nineteen to seventy-three. Moreover, the number of member states that have integrated Traditional Healing training into medical education is also improving. While it notes that 56 per cent of member states have no integration, some 30 per cent do—albeit what is offered ranges from some to a good deal. The other 14 per cent did not answer the question.

There is more good news from this WHO (2013) report. The WHO reports that over one hundred million Europeans are current users of traditional and complementary medicine, with 20 per cent being regular and 20 per cent preferring traditional and complementary medicine. In China, the traditional and complementary medicine market was estimated to be $83.1 billion USD in 2012 (which was a 20 per cent increase from 2011). In addition, the number of traditional and complementary medicine visits in China was 907 million in 2009, some 18 per cent of all medical visits to institutions surveyed. While in the United States, the out-of-pocket expenses for traditional and complementary medicine were $14.8 billion USD in 2008. In Canada, 70 per cent of the population used traditional and complementary medicine in 2012.

The WHO (2013) concludes that cost saving is an important reason to opt for traditional and complementary medicine. Studies show that patients whose general practitioner "has additional complementary and alternative medicine training have lower health care costs and mortality rates than those who do not. Reduced costs were the outcome of fewer hospital stays and fewer prescription drugs" (29). Consequently, the WHO sees such healing systems as part of the tools needed to deliver universal health care coverage. However, many barriers exist. It also makes clear, as noted above, there is no need for traditional and complementary medicine and traditional Western medical systems to clash. In fact, in China, Korea, and Vietnam the one works alongside the second; and Switzerland was the first European country to integrate traditional and complementary medicine into its health care system. However, the WHO insists that integration should follow knowledge-based policies, such as outcome and effectiveness studies, comparative effectiveness research, and patterns of use. Clearly, there is an opportunity to apply research to develop a broad evidence base to inform national policy and decision making—albeit using scientific methods and culture to make judgments on Traditional Knowledge.

The WHO advocates the strategic importance of traditional and complementary medicine, which includes offering low-cost, accessible, and safe health care options for millions of rural households. In addition, Traditional

Knowledge-based healing is important, because of the failure of mainstream medicine to deliver primary health care evenly worldwide. The role of traditional health practitioners in the community health context fills a void in modern health care access. They play a critical complementary role in parallel to the science-based health system. This suggests a multi-pronged policy approach to health care delivery, where various resources need to converge, including those related to local health traditions. This brings us back to a pragmatic point made earlier in the context of protecting Traditional Knowledge that also applies to health care provision: Why not employ all the tools that work, regardless of whence they came? That is, why not use Traditional Healing knowledge and practices alongside medical health knowledge and practices?

NOTES

1. The opinions expressed in this chapter are those of the author and are not necessarily shared by his employer or any other institution with which he is or was associated. At present he is a private scholar.

2. Complementary and alternative medicines in countries like Canada include naturopathy, massage therapy, herbal medications and vitamins, reflexology and chiropractic treatment, and other approaches to healing outside the purview of formal biomedicine.

3. Braiding is discussed in the first chapter of *Knowing Home: Braiding Indigenous Science with Western Science, Book 2*: "'Braiding Indigenous Science and Western Science' is a metaphor used to establish a particular relationship, an obligation of sorts to give, to receive, and to reciprocate. We braid cedar bark to make beautiful baskets, bracelets, and blankets. When braiding hair, kindness and love can flow between the braids. Linked by braiding, there is a certain reciprocity amongst strands, all the strands hold together. Each strand remains a separate entity, a certain tension is required, but all strands come together to form the whole. When we braid Indigenous Science (IS) with Western Science (WS) we acknowledge that both ways of knowing are legitimate forms of knowledge. For Indigenous peoples, Indigenous Knowledge (Indigenous Science) is a gift. It cannot be simply bought and sold. Certain obligations are attached. The more something is shared, the greater becomes its value" (Snively and Williams 2018).

4. See Government of Canada, Indigenous Peoples and Intellectual Property, https://www.ic.gc.ca/eic/site/108.nsf/eng/00004.html.

5. A United Nations multilateral treaty, it is known formally as the Convention on Biological Diversity.

REFERENCES

Agrawal, A. 1993. "Indigenous and Scientific Knowledge: Some Critical Comments."
    Indigenous Knowledge and Development Monitor 3, no. 3: 3–6.

Agrawal, A. 1995. "Dismantling the Divide between Indigenous and Scientific Knowledge."
    Development and Culture 26, no. 3: 413–39. http://www-personal.umich.edu/
    ~arunagra/papers/Dismantling%20the%20Divide.pdf.

Agrawal, A. 2002. *Indigenous Knowledge and the Politics of Classification.* Oxford, UK:
    Blackwell Publishers.

Aguilar, G. 2001. "Access to Genetic Resources and Protection of Traditional Knowledge in
    the Territories of Indigenous Peoples." *Environmental Science and Policy* 4: 241–56.

Alves, R.R.N., and I.M.L. Rosa. 2007. "Biodiversity, Traditional Medicine and Public Health:
    Where Do They Meet?" *Journal of Ethnobiology and Ethnomedicine* 3, no. 14. http://
    www.ethnobiomed.com/content/3/1/14.

Arquette, M., M. Cole, K. Cook, B. LaFrance, M. Peters, J. Ransom, E. Sargent, et al. 2002.
    "Holistic Risk-Based Environmental Decision Making: A Native Perspective."
    Environmental Health Perspective Sup. 2 (April): 259–64.

Balick, M.J., and P.A. Cox. 2021. *Plants, People and Culture: The Science of Ethnobotany.*
    Boca Raton, FL: CRC Press.

Berkes, F. 1999. *Sacred Ecology: Traditional Ecological Knowledge and Resource
    Management.* Philadelphia, PA: Taylor and Francis.

Castellano, M. 2009. "Reflections on Identity and Empowerment: Recurring Themes in the
    Discourse on and with Aboriginal Youth." *Horizons* 10, no. 1: 7–12.

Chandler, M.J., and C.E. Lalonde. 2008. "Cultural Continuity as a Moderator of Suicide
    Risk among Canada's First Nations." In *Healing Traditions: The Mental Health of
    Aboriginal Peoples in Canada,* edited by L. Kirmayer and G. Valaskakis, 221–48.
    Vancouver: UBC Press.

The Crucible Group. 1994. *People, Plants, and Patents: The Impact of Intellectual Property
    on Trade, Plant Biodiversity and Rural Society.* Ottawa: International Development
    Research Centre.

Dirks, N., G. Eley, and S. Ortner, eds. 1994. Introduction to *Culture-Power-History: A Reader
    in Contemporary Social Theory,* 3–45. Princeton: Princeton University Press.

Feyerabend, P. 1975. *Against Method.* London: Verso.

Franklin, S. 1995. "Science as Culture, Cultures of Science." *Annual Review of Anthropology*
    24 (October): 163–84.

Golan, J., S. Athayde, E.A. Olson, and A. McAlvay. 2019. "Intellectual Property Rights and
    Ethnobiology: An Update on Posey's Call to Action." *Journal of Ethnobiology* 39, no. 1:
    90–109.

Government of Bhutan. 2003. *The Biodiversity Act of Bhutan*. World Intellectual Property. http://www.wipo.int/wipolex/en/text.jsp?file_id=168016.

Government of Canada. n.d. *Indigenous Traditional Knowledge and Intellectual Property Rights*. Ottawa: Library of Parliament.

Government of Canada. 2022. *Introduction to Intellectual Property Rights and the Protection of Indigenous Knowledge and Cultural Expressions in Canada*. Innovation, Science and Economic Development Canada. https://www.ic.gc.ca/eic/site/108.nsf/eng/00007.html.

Indigenous and Northern Affairs Canada (INAC)/Government of Canada. 1999. *Intellectual Property and Aboriginal People: A Working Paper*. Ottawa: Minister of Public Works and Government Services Canada. https://publications.gc.ca/collections/Collection/R32-204-1999E.pdf.

International Labor Organization Convention. 1989. Indigenous and Tribal Peoples Convention No. 169. https://www.ilo.org/dyn/normlex/en/f?p=NORMLEX-PUB:55:0::NO::P55_TYPE,P55_LANG,P55_DOCUMENT,P55_NODE:REV,en,C169,/Document.

Kimmerer, R.W. 2002. "Weaving Traditional Ecological Knowledge into Biological Education: A Call to Action." *BioScience* 52, no. 5: 432–38.

Kuhn, T. 1962. *The Structure of Scientific Revolutions*. Chicago: The University of Chicago Press.

LaDuke, W. 1994. "Traditional Ecological Knowledge and Environmental Futures." *Colorado Journal of International Environmental Law and Policy* 5: 127–48.

Legislative Assembly of the Republic of Costa Rica. 1998. Biodiversity Law 7788. https://www.endangeredearth.com/wp-content/uploads/es_laws/Costa-Rica-Biodiversity-Law-of-Costa-Rica.pdf.

Levi-Strauss, C. 1967. *Structural Anthropology*. New York: Doubleday Anchor.

Maffi, L., and E. Woodley. 2010. *Biocultural Diversity Conservation: A Global Sourcebook*. London: Earthscan.

McGonigle, I.V. 2016. "Patenting Nature or Protecting Culture? Ethnopharmacology and Indigenous Intellectual Property Rights." *Journal of Law and the Biosciences* 3, no. 1: 17–226.

McGregor, D. 2008. "Linking Traditional Ecological and Western Science: Aboriginal Perspectives from the 2000 State of the Lakes Conference." *The Canadian Journal of Native Studies* XXVIII, no. 1: 139–58.

Moffa, A. 2016. "Traditional Ecological Rulemaking." *Stanford Environmental Law Journal* 35, no. 2: 101–55.

Mugabe, J. 1999. *Intellectual Property Protection, and Traditional Knowledge: An Exploration in International Policy Discourse*. African Center for Technology Studies.

https://www.wipo.int/edocs/mdocs/tk/en/wipo_unhchr_ip_pnl_98/wipo_unhchr_ip_pnl_98_4.pdf.

National Biodiversity Authority, India. 2013. *People's Biodiversity Registrar.* http://nbaindia.org/uploaded/pdf/PBR%20Format%202013.pdf.

North American Regional Declaration on Biocultural Diversity. 2019. *The Atateken Declaration.* May 2019. https://www.cbd.int/portals/culturaldiversity/docs/north-american-regional-declaration-on-biocultural-diversity-en.pdf.

Posey, D. 1990. "Intellectual Property Rights: And Just Compensation for Indigenous Knowledge." *Anthropology Today* 6, no. 4: 13–16.

Posey, D., and G. Dutfield. 1996. *Beyond Intellectual Property: Toward Traditional Resource Rights for Indigenous Peoples and Local Communities.* Ottawa: International Development Research Centre.

Sciences Act Administration. 1988. *Sciences Act.* Consolidation. R.S.N.W.T, c. S-4. https://nwtresearch.com/research/nwt-research-policies/scientists-act.

Simpson, L. 2001. "Aboriginal Peoples and Knowledge: Decolonizing Our Processes." *Canadian Journal of Native Studies* XXI, no. 1: 137–48.

Simpson, L. 2004. "Anticolonial Strategies for the Recovery and Maintenance of Indigenous Knowledge." *The American Indian Quarterly* 28, nos. 3 & 4: 373–84.

Simpson, L. 1999. "The Construction of Traditional Ecological Knowledge: Issues Implications and Insight." PhD dissertation, University of Manitoba. http://hdl.handle.net/1993/2210.

Snively, G., and Wanosts'a7 L. Williams. 2018. "Braiding Indigenous Science with Western Science." In *Knowing Home: Braiding Indigenous Science with Western Science, Book 2,* edited by G. Snively and L. Williams Wanosts'a7, 3–14. https://pressbooks.bccampus.ca/knowinghome2/.Walking Together FINAL COPYEDIT.docx.

Tauli-Corpuz, V. 2004. *Biodiversity, Traditional Knowledge and Rights of Indigenous Peoples.* Third World Network Berhad, Intellectual Property Rights Series No. 5. https://www.twn.my/title/bioipr.htm.

Tsuji, L.J.S., and E. Ho. 2002. "Traditional Environmental Knowledge and Western Science: In Search of Common Ground." *The Canadian Journal of Native Studies* XXII, no. 2: 327–60.

Tulloch, S. 2009. "Uqausirtinnik Annirusunniq: Longing for Our Language." *Horizons* 10, no. 1: 73–78.

United Nations (UN). 1992. *Convention on Biological Diversity.* https://www.cbd.int/doc/legal/cbd-en.pdf.

United Nations (UN). 2008. *United Nations Declaration on the Rights of Indigenous Peoples.* http://www.un.org/esa/socdev/unpfii/documents/DRIPS_en.pdf.

United Nations (UN). 1948. Universal Declaration of Human Rights. https://www.un.org/
sites/un2.un.org/files/2021/03/udhr.pdf.

United Nations University. 2012. *Biodiversity, Traditional Knowledge and Community
Health: Strengthening the Linkages.* http://archive.ias.unu.edu/resource_centre/
Biodiversity%20Traditional%20Knowledge%20and%20Community%20Health_
final.pdf.

World Health Organization (WHO). 2002. Programme on Traditional Medicine.
WHO Traditional Medicine Strategy 2002–2005. https://apps.who.int/iris/
handle/10665/67163.

World Health Organization (WHO). 2003. *Traditional Medicine.* Fact Sheet No. 134. https://
apps.who.int/gb/ebwha/pdf_files/EB134/B134_24-en.pdf.

World Health Organization (WHO). 2019. *WHO Global Report on Traditional and
Complementary Medicine.* https://www.who.int/traditional-complementary-integra-
tive-medicine/WhoGlobalReportOnTraditionalAndComplementaryMedicine2019.pdf.

World Health Organization (WHO). 2013. *WHO Traditional Medicine Strategy 2014–2023.*
https://www.who.int/publications/i/item/9789241506096.

World Intellectual Property Organization. n.d. Traditional Knowledge. https://www.wipo.
int/tk/en/tk/.

World People's Conference on Climate Change and the Rights of Mother Earth. 2010.
Universal Declaration of Rights of Mother Earth. https://566259-1852283-raikfcquax-
qncofqfm.stackpathdns.com/wp-content/uploads/2021/09/FINAL-UNIVERSAL-
DECLARATION-OF-THE-RIGHTS-OF-MOTHER-EARTH-APRIL-22-2010.pdf.

Wyndham, F.S. 2017. "The Trouble with TEK." *Ethnobiology Letters* 8, no. 1: 78–80.

11   Diabetes and Culture

Time to Truly and Sincerely Listen to Indigenous Peoples

RICHARD T. OSTER, ANGELA GRIER,

RICK LIGHTNING, MARIA J. MAYAN,

AND ELLEN L. TOTH

This chapter's authors have been engaged in important work on diabetes prevention and management in Indigenous communities in Alberta. Given the huge health burden diabetes poses in Indigenous communities, understanding and managing risk factors in culturally feasible ways is a significant undertaking. These researchers and practitioners were invited to contribute to this book because their work exemplifies culturally appropriate collaborative work on Indigenous community health problems.

There is no shortage of literature and research describing the many health conditions that excessively and negatively affect Indigenous Peoples in Canada, and globally. Diabetes, mainly type 2 diabetes, dominates such discussions in that it has exploded over the past three to four decades in many Indigenous Peoples, and its complications wreak havoc in the form of blindness, amputations, dialysis, and early death from cardiovascular disease. Many researchers, policy makers, and funders are attempting to manage and prevent type 2 diabetes, often in collaboration with Indigenous communities and at the impetus of grassroots movements, with the best of intentions. The results of these attempts that have largely been based out of non-Indigenous methodologies and approaches have been modest at best, as far as the numbers can tell us. There continue to be more and more people with diabetes, and the suffering has not abated.

All along the way, Indigenous Peoples have been voicing a message of the link between the loss and destruction of their traditional cultures and ways of life, and the impact of this on their health (e.g., cancer, mental health), and in particular, type 2 diabetes. But have they been heard? We feel they have not. In this chapter, we will discuss the necessity to sincerely listen to this message. First, we provide an overview of the burden of type 2 diabetes and its complications in Indigenous Peoples in Canada, and present some of the notable research collaborations that have addressed this health crisis. Next, we describe a simple model for the underlying causes of type 2 diabetes in Indigenous Peoples in Canada, drawing attention to the fundamental role of colonization and cultural destruction. Finally, we draw on some of our recent work on cultural continuity as we make a case for Indigenous cultural reclamation in the battle against type 2 diabetes.

Type 2 Diabetes Epidemiology in Canadian Indigenous Populations

A seemingly unrelenting global increase in type 2 diabetes is occurring (Shaw, Sicree, and Zimmet et al. 2010). Many Indigenous Peoples around the world have been the hardest hit, experiencing dramatic increases in type 2 diabetes incidence and prevalence, despite their varied experiences, identities, histories, and genetic backgrounds (Yu and Zinman 2007). Indigenous Peoples in Canada (constitutionally recognized as First Nations, Métis, and Inuit) have not been exempt from the type 2 diabetes crisis. Since contact with European settlers and colonization, Indigenous Peoples in Canada have experienced starvation, wars, infectious diseases, and substantial depopulation, with a slow repopulation and a rise in chronic diseases such as obesity, cardiovascular disease, and type 2 diabetes (Waldram, Herring, and Young 2006). In fact, studies continue to report type 2 diabetes rates at least twice as high, and in some cases up to five times as high among Indigenous Peoples compared to the general Canadian population (Dyck et al. 2010; Oster et al. 2011b; Young et al. 2000).

The vast majority of what is known of the epidemiology of type 2 diabetes in Indigenous Peoples in Canada has been determined from First Nations populations. This is in part due to the relative ease of identifying First Nations individuals in administrative databases by their Treaty status. Moreover, First Nations peoples are the largest Indigenous group in Canada and comprise approximately 2.2 per cent of the total population (Statistics Canada 2006). Lillian Chase (1937) reported, now famously, that diabetes was not present in any of a large sample of First Nations peoples in Saskatchewan prior to the 1940s. However, during the 1990s and 2000s, researchers and communities documented an explosion of type 2 diabetes in First Nations peoples. Up-to-date prevalence estimates differ, depending on the methodology used and the specific population being examined, but likely all of these are underestimated due to high rates of undiagnosed type 2 diabetes observed in First Nations peoples (Harris et al. 1997; Oster and Toth 2009).

Selected prevalence rates that have been reported for Indigenous populations in different parts of Canada are depicted in Table 11.1 (one survey is provided for a non-Indigenous comparison group).

TABLE 11.1 *Diabetes Prevalence Rates from Selected Studies*

Author	Method	Location	Population	Prevalence
Statistics Canada (2010)	Age-standardized self-report survey	Canada	General population > 12 years	6.40%
First Nations Information Governance Centre (2011)	Age-standardized self-report survey	Canada	Adult First Nations	20.70%
Harris et al. (1997)	Age- and sex-standardized community screening	Sandy Lake, Ontario	Adult First Nations women	28.00%
			Adult First Nations men	24.20%
Shah, Cauch-Dudek, and Pigeau (2011)	Age-standardized administrative data	Ontario	Adult Métis	11.80%

Author	Method	Location	Population	Prevalence
Horn et al. (2007)	Age-standardized hospital registry/band membership data	Kahnawake, Quebec	Adult First Nations women	7.10%
			Adult First Nations men	8.40%
Dannenbaum et al. (2008)	Age-standardized chart review	Eastern James Bay, Quebec	Adult First Nations	22.40%
Dyck et al. (2010)	Age- and sex-standardized administrative data	Saskatchewan	Adult First Nations women	20.30%
			Adult First Nations men	16.00%
Green et al. (2003)	Age-standardized administrative data	Manitoba	Adult First Nations	20.90%
Martens et al. (2010)	Age-standardized administrative data	Manitoba	Adult Métis	11.20%
Riediger et al. (2014)	Age-standardized population screening	Sandy Bay, Manitoba	Adult First Nations	29.60%
Oster et al. (2011b)	Age-standardized administrative data	Alberta	Adult First Nations	13.50%
Ralph-Campbell et al. (2006)	Age-standardized self-report survey	Alberta	Métis on Settlements	6.90%
Patenaude et al. (2005)	Age-standardized retrospective population-based medical chart review	Bella Coola, British Columbia	Adult Aboriginal	12.50%
Egeland, Cao, and Young (2011)	Weighted population screening	Canadian Arctic	Inuit > 50 years	12.20%
			Inuit < 50 years	1.90%

First Nations females tend to have higher diabetes prevalence rates compared to their male counterparts, which is the reverse of what has been shown in the general Canadian population, where rates are even among both sexes, or even slightly higher for males (Dyck et al. 2010; Oster et al. 2011b). In Saskatchewan, age-adjusted diabetes prevalence was 20.3 per cent for First Nations women and 16.0 per cent for First Nations men in 2005. First Nations peoples in Alberta share similar results (Oster et al. 2011b). However, this sex-specific gap in diabetes may be diminishing as First Nations males experienced a significantly accelerated rise in diabetes prevalence and incidence compared to First Nations females between 1995 and 2007 in Alberta (Oster et al. 2011b). Maternal gestational diabetes and pregestational diabetes[1] is noticeably higher among First Nations women compared to non-First Nations women, likely contributing to the higher type 2 diabetes rates in First Nations women compared to men (Cheung and Byth 2003; Oster et al. 2014b). Finally, type 2 diabetes is affecting First Nations peoples at a younger age than the general Canadian population. In Saskatchewan, the number of incident cases was highest among First Nations adults aged 40–49, whereas most new diabetes cases among the general population were among those greater than seventy years of age (Dyck et al. 2010).

Longitudinal studies suggest that type 2 diabetes will continue to rise in Canadian Indigenous Peoples. Among Alberta Métis Settlements, age-adjusted diabetes prevalence increased from 5.1 per cent in 1998 to 6.9 per cent in 2006 (Ralph-Campbell et al. 2009). The prevalence of diabetes increased between 1980 and 2005, from 9.5 per cent to 20.3 per cent among First Nations women, and from 4.9 per cent to 16.0 per cent among First Nations men in Saskatchewan (Dyck et al. 2010). Although significant increases in the prevalence and incidence of diabetes from 1995 to 2007 were also reported for the adult First Nations population in Alberta, the increase was less pronounced in the First Nations population than in the general population (Oster et al. 2011b). In Saskatchewan, age-adjusted diabetes prevalence among First Nations youth more than tripled from 71.2/100,000 and 70.0/100,000 for girls and boys, respectively, in 1980–1981 to 230.1/100,000 and 196.6/100,000 in 2003–2005 (Dyck et al. 2012). Similarly in Alberta, diabetes prevalence grew among First

Nations youth at a rate almost twice that of the non-First Nations youth population over a twelve-year time span (Oster et al. 2012).

First Nations peoples with type 2 diabetes have been shown to experience more complications than non-First Nations populations. The national CIRCLE study of 885 randomly sampled First Nations patients with type 2 diabetes found alarmingly high rates of complications and co-morbidities: 92.6 per cent had dyslipidemia, 92.0 per cent had hypertension, 92.1 per cent were overweight or obese, 55.1 per cent had chronic kidney disease, 13.3 per cent had coronary artery disease, 10.8 per cent had neuropathy, 10.7 per cent had retinopathy, and 5.5 per cent had diabetic foot disease (Harris et al. 2011). Rates of undiagnosed complications of type 2 diabetes among First Nations patients in Alberta are substantial: 23 per cent kidney damage, 22 per cent hypercholesterolemia, 11 per cent foot complications, 9 per cent hypertension, and 7 per cent retinopathy (Oster et al. 2009). This increased burden of diabetes is also supported by reports of higher numbers of diabetes-related emergency department and general practitioner visits, as well as longer hospital stays due to diabetes among First Nations compared to non-First Nations (Oster et al. 2011a). In British Columbia, 18 per cent and 21 per cent of deaths among First Nations men and women, respectively, were found to be due to diabetes and its complications (Jin, Martin, and Sarin 2002). Recently, an analysis of national census data showed the relative risk of death due to diabetes was 4.3 times higher for First Nations men and 7.9 times higher for First Nations women compared to their non-First Nations counterparts (Park et al. 2015). In addition, all-cause mortality is 1.6 times higher among First Nations with diabetes than the general population with the disease in Alberta (Oster et al. 2011b). A glimmer of hope from the Alberta data is that mortality rates among those First Nations adults with diabetes has decreased significantly over time (Oster et al. 2011b).

Notable Research Collaborations Addressing Type 2 Diabetes
in Indigenous Populations in Canada

It is clear from these grim statistics that type 2 diabetes continues to disproportionately impact Indigenous Peoples in Canada. There has been an apparent response to this diabetes crisis, including the federally funded Aboriginal Diabetes Initiative, and diverse interventions and programs from community-based prevention to complications screening. In Table 11.2 we present a summary of some of the major Canadian efforts to prevent or manage type 2 diabetes specific to Indigenous populations, with estimated or published outcomes. Of note, a systematic worldwide literature search of publications on diabetes affecting Indigenous populations between 2006 and 2011 on the occasion of drafting the 2013 Canadian Clinical Practice Guidelines revealed 235 high-quality references, with forty-nine by Canadian authors. Of these forty-nine, ten concerned basic science, fifteen were epidemiological reports, eighteen described complications and burden of diabetes, two discussed prevention, and six described attempts at improving management. Prevention and management efforts being typically the most costly and difficult to undertake, they are likely under-represented in the literature, either because they are not occurring or they are not succeeding.

TABLE 11.2 *Major Canadian Efforts to Prevent or Manage Type 2 Diabetes Specific to Indigenous Populations*

Author/Location/ Population	Description of Prevention or Management
Aboriginal Diabetes Initiative (1999–2015) / Canada / predominantly First Nations on reserve, Métis, off-reserve First Nations, and urban Inuit	"Established in 1999, the Aboriginal Diabetes Initiative (ADI) had initial funding of $58 million over five years. It was then expanded in 2005 with a budget of $190 million over five years. Currently [to 2015], Health Canada is investing over $50 million per year to support the third phase, as the government continues supporting health promotion and diabetes prevention activities and services" (Government of Canada).

Author/Location/ Population	Description of Prevention or Management
	"A wide range of community-led and culturally relevant health promotion and prevention activities have been offered in over 600 First Nations and Inuit communities to promote diabetes awareness, healthy eating and physical activity as part of healthy lifestyles" (Government of Canada).
	"Mobile diabetes screening initiatives have been held in four regions (British Columbia, Alberta, Manitoba and Quebec). In other regions, screening is carried out through local health-care providers. Some communities have formed partnerships with neighboring provincial healthcare services to increase screening opportunities" (Government of Canada). "Supported the Canadian First Nations Diabetes Clinical Management Epidemiologic (CIRCLE) study to determine the quality of diabetes health care in nineteen First Nations communities" (Government of Canada).
	"Supported a component for Métis, Off-reserve Aboriginal and Urban Inuit Promotion and Prevention (MOAUIPP), which provided time-limited, proposal-based funding for culturally relevant diabetes prevention and health promotion projects for these Aboriginal populations. Sixty-six projects were funded between 2006 and 2010" (Government of Canada).
Potvin et al. (2003) / Khanawake, Quebec / First Nations	Research evidence: Dr. Macaulay and her colleagues have published numerous papers that illustrate how to implement participatory research projects in which the end users work in equal partnership with the academic investigators throughout the gathering, analysis, dissemination, and application of knowledge.
Ralph-Campbell et al. (2006) / Alberta / self-identified Aboriginal	Controlled trial of academic marketing to change outcomes in communities. The intervention was associated with a significant improvement in blood pressure (42 per cent intervention vs. 25 per cent control). However, there were only small, nonsignificant changes in cholesterol or hemoglobin A1c. The intervention was associated with a significant increase in satisfaction with diabetes care. Aboriginal participants did not differ in most results from non-Aboriginals but reported worse health-related quality of life.

Author/Location/ Population	Description of Prevention or Management
Tobe et al. (2006) / Saskatchewan / First Nations	Diabetes Risk Evaluation and Microalbuminuria (DREAM 3) randomized controlled trial. Compared intervention strategy (home care nurse following algorithm) and control strategy (treatment decisions made by each subject's primary care physician) for controlling hypertension in First Nations people with hypertension and diabetes. Intervention had a significantly larger decrease in diastolic blood pressure over time than control.
Ho et al. (2006) / Sandy Lake, Ontario / First Nations	In-depth interviews and a structured survey, demonstration and feedback sessions, group activities, and meetings with key stakeholders in communities to find the needs of communities and feedback on prevention interventions (e.g., walking trails).
Ho et al. (2008) / Ontario / First Nations	Prevention of risk factors for diabetes in seven northwestern Ontario First Nations via nine-month lifestyle intervention program in schools, stores, and communities. "Knowledge" and healthy food acquisition improved. There were no significant changes in physical activity or body mass index in either intervention or comparison groups.
Rose et al. (2008) / Ontario / Aboriginal and non-Aboriginal	A retrospective review of medical records was done for 325 patients receiving care during a two-year period. There were 224 (69 per cent) non-Aboriginal and 101 (31 per cent) Aboriginal patients with 697 foot ulcers. A multidisciplinary diabetic foot clinic may be successful in treating diabetic foot ulcers in Aboriginal and non-Aboriginal people. However, the frequency of poor outcome is high, consistent with the high prevalence of associated significant risk factors in this population.
Ralph-Campbell et al. (2009) / Alberta / off-reserve Aboriginal and Métis Settlements	The Mobile Diabetes Screening Initiative travelled to rural Aboriginal and other remote communities in Alberta to screen for diabetes and cardiovascular risk, education, and community-based care. Among those without diabetes (N = 629), body mass index and weight increased and blood pressure decreased significantly. For those with diabetes (N = 180), significant improvements were observed for all indicators, except waist circumference.

Author/Location/ Population	Description of Prevention or Management
Tobe et al. (2010) / Saskatchewan / First Nations	Diabetes Risk Evaluation and Microalbuminuria (DREAM 3) randomized controlled trial follow-up. The participants that agreed to follow up maintained their blood pressure control and did not revert to baseline levels. Target blood pressure was achieved in 53 per cent of participants.
Oster et al. (2010) / Alberta / First Nations	Diabetes complications screening, diabetes education, and community-based care were provided by mobile clinics that travelled to Alberta First Nations communities. Significant improvements in body mass index, blood pressure, total cholesterol, and hemoglobin A1c concentrations were identified ($p < 0.01$) in subjects who followed up. Significant decreasing secular trends in total cholesterol and hemoglobin A1c concentrations at presentation were observed ($p < 0.01$) over time.
Harris et al. (2011) / James Bay, Quebec / Cree First Nations	Chart review showed room for improvement in diabetes care among First Nations in northern Quebec (Eeyou Istchee): reasonable management of glucose but poor management of complications.
Canadian Institutes of Health Research (2013) / Khanawake, Quebec / First Nations	Evidence in action: Both Kahnawake elementary schools have incorporated a culturally appropriate ten-week course on the importance of healthy eating and physical activity in their curricula, and have implemented healthy nutrition policies. The program supports dozens of recurring interventions— food-tasting sessions to promote healthy/traditional cooking, empowerment workshops, and walking, cycling, and bowling events—to mobilize the community to reduce the incidence of diabetes.
Diabetes Integration Project (2015) / Manitoba / First Nations	The Diabetes Integration Project is an integrated diabetes health care service developed to address the needs of First Nations people who have diabetes. The project is ongoing, and utilizes mobile diabetes health care teams to provide diabetes care and treatment services in First Nations communities throughout Manitoba.

The true impact of these projects is very difficult to ascertain, often due to the lack of proper control groups and a lack of markers of success. Confounding the results are updated clinical practice guidelines, advances in diabetes treatments, federal and provincial initiatives, grassroots and community initiatives, awareness campaigns, changing socio-economic environments, and other intangibles, all of which could have had an influence, making it unclear why particular efforts made an impact. What is clear is that type 2 diabetes is still exceptionally common in Indigenous Peoples in Canada, and the critical need for programs and interventions has not dissipated.

A Model for the Causes of Type 2 Diabetes in Indigenous Populations in Canada

With the type 2 diabetes crisis still raging, it is important to understand where previous efforts have been targeted, and where we might target new efforts. To do so requires a model of the causation of type 2 diabetes, a daunting task given the complexity of the disease. A massive amount of work over the past few decades has been dedicated to understanding the intricate and multi-faceted risk factors, mechanisms, etiology, and patho-physiology of type 2 diabetes. An important Canadian effort continues to target biological, genetic, and contextual predictors of chronic disease, including diabetes and cancer (Montreal Heart Institute 2015). However, the differential risk in Indigenous Peoples is as yet unaccounted for. Increasingly, the social determinants of health are being touted as the "causes of the causes," and while genetic predisposition and biological markers may be of interest, it seems to be determinants like income and education levels, and access to safe housing and clean water that determine the impact of diabetes (and other chronic diseases) the most (Braveman, Egerter, and Williams 2011).

In this section, we present a simple model for specifically understanding type 2 diabetes in Indigenous populations in Canada to determine where we might target our efforts (Figure 11.1). This model is based on three areas of knowledge: the extant literature on type 2 diabetes in Indigenous Peoples, our own research in diabetes and experience working with Indigenous communities, and written and oral accounts from Indigenous Peoples.

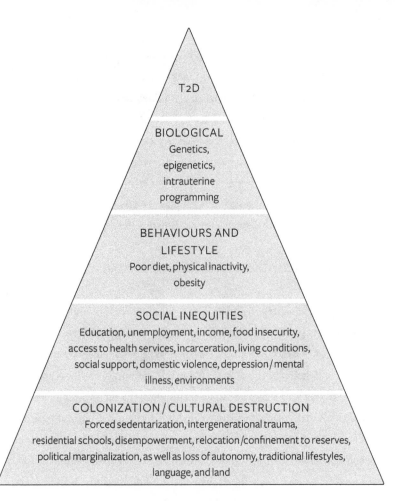

FIGURE 11.1 *Model for the causes of type 2 diabetes in Canadian Indigenous populations.*

We feel this model helps to visualize type 2 diabetes as the "tip of the iceberg," and a symptom of inequities in the social determinants of health, all underpinned by colonization and cultural destruction.

There is little doubt that type 2 diabetes is being driven predominately by poor diet, sedentary behaviours, and resultant overweight and obesity (Hu et al. 2001), all of which are significantly more prevalent among Indigenous Peoples in Canada (Bryan et al. 2006; First Nations Information Governance Centre 2011; Willows 2005). How lifestyle and environmental exposures interact with genes through epigenetic changes—particularly during the prenatal period and early life—also plays an important role in the risk for type 2 diabetes (Mendelson et al. 2011), as does genetic predispositions (Pollex et al. 2005). However, to stop there would be very short-sighted, and would perpetuate damaging and negative stereotypes. We need to dig deeper than that to ask, "What are the causes of the causes?"

Many Indigenous Peoples have lower completion rates of all levels of education, higher unemployment rates, lower incomes, higher food insecurity rates, poorer quality and poorer access to health services, higher rates of criminal activity and incarceration, more crowded and dilapidated living conditions, less social support, higher rates of domestic violence, and higher rates of depression and mental illness (Adelson 2005; King, Smith, and Gracey 2009). The connections between these social determinants of health and conditions such as type 2 diabetes are well known (Hill, Nielsen, and Fox 2013; Whiting, Unwinm, and Roglic 2010). But why, in a First World nation, are there such dramatic social disparities for Canadian Indigenous Peoples? It is the continued colonization efforts and the cultural attacks by the "mainstream" or dominant population.

Indigenous Peoples in Canada have been subject to frequent and numerous cultural and evolutionary disturbances, including (but not limited to) the decimation of traditional lifestyles, forced sedentarization, intergenerational trauma and residential school, loss of language, disempowerment, political marginalization, loss of autonomy, systemic racism, relocation/confinement to reserves and the loss of land (and connection to the land), as well as emotional, spiritual, and mental disconnection (Gracey and King 2009; King, Smith, and Gracey 2009). The lived realities for Indigenous Peoples today are directly being impacted by racialized legislation, assimilation practices, and archaic and diminished relations between their community leaders and the powers that be politically. Indigenous Peoples have been impacted through continual violence projected at them from the dominant government, and the outcomes are evident that their health is impacted significantly. Thus, Indigenous Peoples are disempowered when it comes to the tools that might work to minimize the gap in social inequities (King, Smith, and Gracey 2009; Reading and Wien 2009).

When we consider our model (Figure 11.1), we can see that most of the research work aimed at preventing and managing type 2 diabetes has intervened predominantly at the behaviours and lifestyle level, or higher in the pyramid, and to a lesser degree at the social inequities level. This has largely been from a paternalistic approach common to a colonial model. However, only now is the clinical and research community becoming aware that Indigenous Peoples must be participants in their own lives, as they always should have. To our knowledge, there have been no type 2 diabetes research programs or interventions that have targeted colonization and cultural destruction deliberately and specifically. Culture and cultural sensitivity are often included in research designs, as they should be, but have yet to be the focus.

Indigenous Cultural Reclamation in the Battle against Type 2 Diabetes
The notion of culture and health being inseparably linked is nothing new to Indigenous Peoples. This is something they have known for time immemorial (Gracey and King 2009). Indigenous Peoples, community members, leaders, Elders, scholars, writers, and so on have emphasized the crucial importance of a strong connection to culture when it comes to health and well-being. Culture is health, and the two cannot be segregated (Oster et al. 2014a). Also, the collective educated and informed knowledge of Indigenous Peoples heard via the Royal Commission on Aboriginal Peoples, the Truth and Reconciliation Commission, Idle No More, and other movements also clearly shows cultural reclamation as imperative to improving or recapturing Indigenous health. Type 2 diabetes is no exception. Furthermore, the root cause of not only type 2 diabetes but many of the contemporary health issues that Indigenous Peoples face is increasingly speculated to be a result of cultural and spiritual loss and colonization (Gracey and King 2009; Hunter et al. 2006; King, Smith, and Gracey 2009; Kirmayer, Simpson, and Cargo 2003), with some evidence provided by the influential and often cited work of Chandler and Lalonde.

Chandler and Lalonde (1998, 2003) utilized both publicly available data and government mortality data on First Nations communities in British Columbia to show that youth suicide rates differed considerably, conditional on the level of community "cultural continuity" (defined as contemporary preservation of traditional culture). In particular, an inverse relationship was found between youth suicide rates and cultural continuity: decreased suicide rates were related to a strong sense of identity among youth, and explained through increased community cultural continuity (Chandler and Lalonde 1998, 2003). Subsequently, reconnection with and revitalization of traditional culture has been a successful strategy to combat alcohol and substance abuse in several First Nations communities by increasing self-esteem, social support, and community connection (McCormick 2000). The Santé Quebec Cree health survey found that more time reported spent in the bush practising traditional hunting/gathering activities was associated with decreased distress (Kirmayer et al. 2000). Also, teenage First Nations males at high risk for suicide reported increased cultural pride, positive cultural identity, as well as pro-social and cooperative behaviours as a result of organized traditional activities in a wilderness setting (Janelle, Laliberte, and Ottawa 2009). Despite these positive results in mental health research, very little work has extrapolated culture as a protective factor to other health issues, such as type 2 diabetes.

In the mid-1990s, type 2 diabetes prevalence was found to be lower among remote First Nations communities in Saskatchewan with less exposure to non-Indigenous lifestyles (Dyck, Tan, and Hoeppner 1995; Pioro, Dyck, and Gillis 1996), with the authors speculating that Euro-Western acculturation may increase diabetes risk. *The Alberta Diabetes Atlas* lends support to this premise, as First Nations prevalence rates in the remote northern regions of the province were lower than the provincial average for the First Nations population (Oster et al. 2011a). Furthermore, much qualitative work has illuminated the underlying role of cultural destruction and colonization of Indigenous Peoples in Canada with type 2 diabetes (Barton, Anderson, and Thommasen 2005; Bruyere and Garro 2000; Garro 1995; Ghosh 2012). We recently set out to provide quantitative evidence by examining the impact of cultural continuity and type 2 diabetes risk among First Nations communities in Alberta (Oster et al. 2014a).

Our work began by interviewing First Nations leaders in an attempt to better understand cultural continuity, what it entails, and how it may be related to health and type 2 diabetes. Qualitative analyses revealed unvaryingly that, without a strong connection to traditional culture, and having that culture continue into future generations, healthy First Nations peoples and communities cannot exist. In other words, culture is the blueprint for healthy First Nations. During the interviews, loss of culture was repeatedly described as the root cause of type 2 diabetes. Similarly, reclamation of culture was described as the solution to type 2 diabetes, as it would act to stabilize communities in troublesome times, to enhance and preserve their shared identity, to build social support, to promote healthy interpersonal relationships, to deliver spiritual tranquillity, to allow for increased physical activity and healthy eating through traditional activities, and ultimately to provide real and effective strategies for living, surviving, and being well. Leaders expressed to us that First Nations have been fighting, and will continue to fight, to reclaim their culture, with the end goal of health and well-being for their communities (Oster et al. 2014a). So, in that sense, many Indigenous communities are already "intervening" at the colonization/ cultural destruction level.

Encouraged by the stories we heard from First Nations leaders, we set out to examine if quantitative evidence would support their claims in fashion similar to that used by Chandler and Lalonde (1998, 2003). Using a cross-sectional approach, we obtained provincial administrative data on diabetes rates and publicly available data on traditional language knowledge rates for thirty-one First Nations communities. We used the language knowledge rates as a proxy measure of cultural continuity (supported by our qualitative research described above). We were also able to obtain median household income, unemployment rates, and high school completion rates to control for socio-economic differences. We found crude diabetes prevalence varied radically among First Nations, with values as low as 1.2 per cent and as high as 18.3 per cent. Likewise, traditional language knowledge prevalence was strikingly different between communities with a low of 10.5 per cent and a high of 92.8 per cent. After adjusting for socio-economic factors, we found an inverse relationship between cultural continuity (measured by traditional Indigenous language knowledge) and diabetes prevalence in regression analysis ($p = 0.007$) (see Figure 11.2). Thus, cultural continuity and reclaiming culture may be protective against type 2 diabetes (Oster et al. 2014a). It is

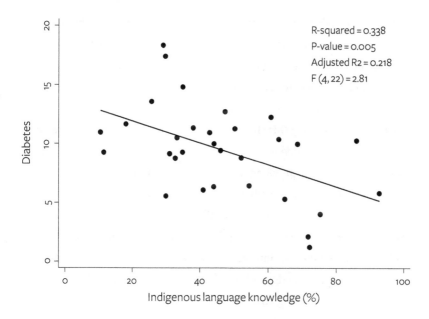

FIGURE 11.2 *Crude diabetes prevalence by Indigenous language knowledge rates for the year 2005.*

our hope that the findings of our research provide the evidence needed for Indigenous Peoples and communities, as well as research programs, to further advocate for and work toward cultural reclamation as a means to reduce the burden of type 2 diabetes.

Conclusion

The cornerstone of effective research interventions and programs with Indigenous Peoples is, and will continue to be, mutual collaboration between researchers and Indigenous communities (Canadian Institutes of Health Research, Natural Sciences and Engineering Research Council of Canada, and Social Sciences and Humanities Research Council of Canada 2018). Many research programs and interventions aimed at type 2 diabetes have done well to include Indigenous stakeholders and community members, and even to include traditional Indigenous culture in many instances. However, to our knowledge, attempts to collaborate with communities to tackle the root causes of diabetes that stem from the effects of colonization have yet to be done. It is not enough to simply conduct research in a "culturally sensitive way." We need to start engaging in Indigenous methodology of research, where the practice is practical and localized, rather than removed and without investment, and we need to make culture the focus.

Our intent in writing this chapter is not to point the finger or place blame. If that were the case, then we would most certainly be blaming ourselves. Rather, our intent is to provide further rationale to design interventions and research studies that specifically address cultural reclamation as a means of fighting diabetes among Indigenous Peoples. While it is true that good diabetes-related surveillance work, primary health care work, epigenetic work, systems and lifestyle intervention work, and so forth are useful and must continue, we argue that cultural reclamation has the potential to reverse some of the lasting effects of colonization on Indigenous Peoples in Canada, and subsequently have an impact on the social determinants of health, lifestyle, and ultimately diabetes risk.

Indigenous Peoples have long ago understood the inseparable link between cultural reclamation and health. It is time that individuals who make decisions that affect the lives of Indigenous Peoples finally understand too. Indigenous Peoples are suffering and dying. Many of those people are not a priority for this society. They are attempting to maintain their Indigenous selves, communities, and ways of being in a time and place that tells them continually they cannot. Addressing cultural reclamation tells them they can.

NOTE

1.   Since type 2 diabetes affects Indigenous women at an earlier age, many are in child-bearing age.

REFERENCES

Adelson, N. 2005. "The Embodiment of Inequity: Health Disparities in Aboriginal Canada." *Canadian Journal of Public Health* 96, Supplement 2: S45–61.

Barton, S.S., N. Anderson, and H.V. Thommasen. 2005. "The Diabetes Experiences of Aboriginal People Living in a Rural Canadian Community." *Australian Journal of Rural Health* 13, no. 4: 242–46.

Braveman, P., S. Egerter, and D.R. Williams. 2011. "The Social Determinants of Health: Coming of Age." *Annual Review of Public Health* 32: 381–98.

Bruyere, J., and L.C. Garro. 2000. "'He travels in the body': Nehinaw (Cree) Understandings of Diabetes." *Canadian Nurse* 96, no. 6: 25–28.

Bryan, S.N., M.S. Tremblay, C.E. Perez, C.I. Ardern, and P.T. Katzmarzyk. 2006. "Physical Activity and Ethnicity: Evidence from the Canadian Community Health Survey." *Canadian Journal of Public Health* 97: 271–76.

Canadian Institutes of Health Research. 2013. "A Community Effort: Proving the Power of Participatory Research." *Show Me the Evidence* 1, no. 4 (Spring). https://cihr-irsc.gc.ca/e/documents/show_me_evidence_v1_I4_e.pdf.

Canadian Institutes of Health Research, Natural Sciences and Engineering Research Council of Canada, and Social Sciences and Humanities Research Council of Canada. 2018. "Research Involving the First Nations, Inuit and Métis Peoples of Canada." In *Ethical Conduct for Research Involving Humans*, Chapter 9. Tri-Council Policy Statement. https://ethics.gc.ca/eng/tcps2-eptc2_2018_chapter9-chapitre9.html.

Chandler, M.J., and C. Lalonde. 1998. Cultural Continuity as a Hedge against Suicide in Canada's First Nations." *Transcultural Psychiatry* 35, no. 2: 191–219.

Chandler, M.J., and C. Lalonde. 2003. "Cultural Continuity as a Protective Factor against Suicide in First Nations Youth." *Horizons—A Special Issue on Aboriginal Youth, Hope or Heartbreak: Aboriginal Youth and Canada's Future* 10, no. 1: 68–72.

Chase, L.A. 1937. "The Trend of Diabetes in Saskatchewan, 1905–1934." *Canadian Medical Association Journal* 36, no. 4: 366–69.

Cheung, N.W., and K. Byth. 2003. "Population Health Significance of Gestational Diabetes." *Diabetes Care* 26, no. 7: 2005–9.

Dannenbaum, D., E. Kuzmina, P. Lejeune, J. Torrie, and M. Gangbe. 2008. "Prevalence of Diabetes and Diabetes-related Complications in First Nations Communities in Northern Quebec (Eeyou Istchee), Canada." *Canadian Journal of Diabetes* 32, no. 1: 46–52.

Diabetes Integration Project. 2015. http://diabetesintegrationproject.ca/.

Dyck, R.F., L. Tan, and V.H. Hoeppner. 1995. "Body Mass Index, Gestational Diabetes and Diabetes Mellitus in Three Northern Saskatchewan Aboriginal Communities." *Chronic Diseases in Canada* 16: 24–26.

Dyck, R., N. Osgood, A. Gao, and M.R. Stang. 2012. "The Epidemiology of Diabetes Mellitus among First Nations and non-First Nations Children in Saskatchewan." *Canadian Journal of Diabetes* 36, no. 1: 19–24.

Dyck, R., N. Osgood, T.H. Lin, A. Gao, and M.R. Stang. 2010. "Epidemiology of Diabetes Mellitus among First Nations and non-First Nations Adults." *Canadian Medical Association Journal* 182, no. 3: 249–56.

Egeland, G.M., Z. Cao, and T.K. Young. 2011. "Hypertriglyceridemic-waist Phenotype and Glucose Intolerance among Canadian Inuit: the International Polar Year Inuit Health Survey for Adults 2007–2008." *Canadian Medical Association Journal* 183, no. 9: E553–59.

First Nations Information Governance Centre. 2011. *First Nations Regional Health Survey: RHS Phase 2 (2008/2010) Preliminary Results*. Ottawa: First Nations Information Governance Centre.

Garro, L.C. 1995. "Individual or Societal Responsibility? Explanations of Diabetes in an Anishinaabe (Ojibway) Community." *Social Science & Medicine* 40, no. 1: 37–46.

Ghosh, H. 2012. "Urban Reality of Type 2 Diabetes among First Nations of Eastern Ontario: Western Science and Indigenous Perceptions." *Journal of Global Citizenship and Equity Education* 2, no. 2: 158–81.

Government of Canada. Aboriginal Diabetes Initiative. https://www.sac-isc.gc.ca/eng/15699 60595332/1569960634063.

Gracey, M., and M. King. 2009. "Indigenous Health Part 1: Determinants and Disease Patterns." *Lancet* 374, no. 9683: 65–75.

Green, C., J.F. Blanchard, T.K. Young, and J. Griffith. 2003. "The Epidemiology of Diabetes in the Manitoba-registered First Nation Population: Current Patterns and Comparative Trends." *Diabetes Care* 26, no. 7: 1993–98.

Harris, S.B., J. Gittelsohn, A. Hanley, A. Barnie, T.M. Wolever, J. Gao, et al. 1997. "The Prevalence of NIDDM and Associated Risk Factors in Native Canadians." *Diabetes Care* 20, no. 2: 185–87.

Harris, S.B., M. Naqshbandi, O. Bhattacharyya, A.J. Hanley, J.G. Esler, B. Zinman, and CIRCLE Study Group. 2011. "Major Gaps in Diabetes Clinical Care among Canada's First Nations: Results of the CIRCLE Study." *Diabetes Research and Clinical Practice* 92, no. 2: 272–79.

Hill, J., M. Nielsen, and M.H. Fox. 2013. "Understanding the Social Factors That Contribute to Diabetes: A Means to Informing Health Care and Social Policies for the Chronically Ill." *The Permanente Journal* 17, no. 2: 67–72.

Ho, L.S., J. Gittelsohn, R. Rimal, M.S. Treuth, S. Sharma, A. Rosecrans, and S.B. Harris. 2008. "An Integrated Multi-institutional Diabetes Prevention Program Improves Knowledge and Healthy Food Acquisition in Northwestern Ontario First Nations." *Health Education & Behavior* 35, no. 4: 561–73.

Ho, L.S., J. Gittelsohn, S.B. Harris, and E. Ford. 2006. "Development of an Integrated Diabetes Prevention Program with First Nations in Canada." *Health Promotion International* 21, no. 2: 88–97.

Horn, O.K., H. Jacobs-Whyte, A. Ing, A. Bruegl, G. Paradis, and A.C. Macaulay. 2007. "Incidence and Prevalence of Type 2 Diabetes in the First Nation Community of Kahnawá:ke, Quebec, Canada, 1986–2003." *Canadian Journal of Public Health* 98, no. 6: 438–43.

Hu, F.B., J.E. Manson, M.J. Stampfer, G. Colditz, S. Liu, C.G. Solomon, and W.C. Willett. 2001. "Diet, Lifestyle, and the Risk of Type 2 Diabetes Mellitus in Women." *New England Journal of Medicine* 345: 790–97.

Hunter, L.M., J. Logan, J.G. Goulet, and S. Barton. 2006. "Aboriginal Healing: Regaining Balance and Culture." *Journal of Transcultural Nursing* 17: 13–22.

Janelle, A., A. Laliberte, and U. Ottawa. 2009. "Promoting Traditions: An Evaluation of a Wilderness Activity among First Nations of Canada." *Australasian Psychiatry* 17, Supplement 1: S108–11.

Jin, A., J.D. Martin, and C. Sarin. 2002. "A Diabetes Mellitus in the First Nations Population of British Columbia, Canada, Part 1: Mortality." *International Journal of Circumpolar Health* 61, no. 3: 251–53.

King, M., A. Smith, and M. Gracey. 2009. "Indigenous Health Part 2: The Underlying Causes of the Health Gap." *Lancet* 374, no. 9683: 76–85.

Kirmayer, L.J., C. Simpson, and M. Cargo. 2003. "Healing Traditions: Culture, Community and Mental Health Promotion with Canadian Aboriginal Peoples." *Australasian Psychiatry* 11: S15–23.

Kirmayer, L.J., L.J. Boothroyd, A. Tanner, N. Adelson, and E. Robinson. 2000. "Psychological Distress among the Cree of James Bay." *Transcultural Psychiatry* 37: 35–56.

Martens, P.J., J. Bartlett, E. Burland, H. Prior, C. Burchill, S. Huq, S. Rompf, et al. 2010. *Profile of Métis Health Status and Healthcare Utilization in Manitoba: A Population-Based Study.* Winnipeg: Manitoba Centre for Health Policy.

McCormick, R.M. 2000. "Aboriginal Traditions in the Treatment of Substance Abuse." *Canadian Journal of Counselling* 34: 25–32.

Mendelson, M., J. Cloutier, L. Spence, E. Sellers, S. Taback, and H. Dean. 2011. "Obesity and Type 2 Diabetes Mellitus in a Birth Cohort of First Nation Children Born to Mothers with Pediatric-onset Type 2 Diabetes." *Pediatric Diabetes* 12, no. 3: 219–28.

Montreal Heart Institute. 2015. *A Pan-Canadian, Multi-ethnic Cohort Study in Healthy Participants Aimed to Better Understand the Impact of Individual, Socioeconomic and Other Environmental Factors Leading to Cardiac and Vascular Disease.* Bethesda, MD: National Library of Medicine. https://clinicaltrials.gov/ct2/show/ NCT02220582.

Oster, R.T., A. Grier, R. Lightning, M.J. Mayan, and E.L. Toth. 2014a. "Cultural Continuity, Traditional Indigenous Language, and Diabetes in Alberta First Nations: A Mixed Methods Study." *International Journal for Equity in Health* 13, no. 92. https://equityhealthj.biomedcentral.com/articles/10.1186/s12939-014-0092-4.

Oster, R.T., B.R. Hemmelgarn, E.L. Toth, M. King, and L. Crowshoe. 2011a. "Diabetes and the Status Aboriginal Population in Alberta." In *Alberta Diabetes Atlas 2011*, 177–202. Edmonton: Institute of Health Economics. pdf.https://www.ihe.ca/download/alberta_diabetes_atlas_2011.pdf.

Oster, R.T., and E.L. Toth. 2009. "Differences in the Prevalence of Diabetes Risk-Factors among First Nation, Métis and non-Aboriginal Adults Attending Screening Clinics in Rural Alberta, Canada." *Rural and Remote Health* 9: 1170. https://doi.org/10.22605/RRH1170.

Oster, R.T., J.A. Johnson, B.R. Hemmelgarn, M. King, S.U. Balko, L.W. Svenson, L. Crowshoe, et al. 2011b. "Recent Epidemiologic Trends of Diabetes Mellitus among Status Aboriginal Adults." *Canadian Medical Association Journal* 183, no. 12: E803–08.

Oster, R.T., J.A. Johnson, S.U. Balko, L.W. Svenson, and E.L. Toth. 2012. "Increasing Rates of Diabetes amongst Status Aboriginal Youth in Alberta, Canada." *International Journal of Circumpolar Health* 71: 1–7.

Oster, R.T., M. King, D.W. Morrish, M.J. Mayan, and E.L. Toth. 2014b. "Diabetes in Pregnancy among First Nations Women in Alberta, Canada: A Retrospective Analysis." *BMC Pregnancy and Childbirth* 14, no. 136. https://pubmed.ncbi.nlm.nih.gov/24716718/.

Oster, R.T., S. Shade, D. Strong, and E.L. Toth. 2010. "Improvements in Indicators of Diabetes-Related Health Status among First Nations Individuals Enrolled in a Community-Driven Diabetes Complications Mobile Screening Program in Alberta, Canada." *Canadian Journal of Public Health* 101, no. 5: 410–14.

Oster, R.T., S. Virani, D. Strong, S. Shade, and E.L. Toth. 2009. "Diabetes Care and Health Status of First Nations Individuals with Type 2 Diabetes in Alberta." *Canadian Family Physician* 55, no. 4: 386–593.

Park, J., M. Tjepkema, N. Goedhuis, and P. Pennock. 2015. *Avoidable Mortality among First Nations Adults in Canada: A Cohort Analysis*. Ottawa: Statistics Canada.

Patenaude, J., H.D. Tildesley, A.C. MacArthur, D.C. Voaklander, and H. Thommasen. 2005. "Prevalence of Diabetes Mellitus in Aboriginal and non-Aboriginal People Living in the Bella Coola Valley." *British Columbia Medical Journal* 47, no. 8: 429–37.

Pioro, M., R.F. Dyck, and D.C. Gillis. 1996. "Diabetes Prevalence Rates among First Nations Adults on Saskatchewan Reserves in 1990: Comparison by Tribal Grouping, Geography and with non-First Nation people." *Canadian Journal of Public Health* 87, no. 5: 325–28.

Pollex, R.L., A.J. Hanley, B. Zinman, S.B. Harris, H.M. Khan, and R.A. Hegele. 2005. "Synergism between Mutant HNF1A and the Metabolic Syndrome in Oji-Cree Type 2 Diabetes." *Diabetic Medicine* 22, no. 11: 1510–15.

Potvin, L., M. Cargo, A.M. McComber, T. Delormier, and A.C. Macaulay. 2003. "Implementing Participatory Intervention and Research in Communities: Lessons from the Kahnawake Schools Diabetes Prevention Project in Canada." *Social Science & Medicine* 56, no. 6: 1295–1305.

Ralph-Campbell, K., R.T. Oster, T. Connor, M. Pick, S. Pohar, P. Thompson, M. Daniels, et al. 2009. "Increasing Rates of Diabetes and Cardiovascular Risk in Métis Settlements in Northern Alberta." *International Journal of Circumpolar Health* 68, no. 5: 433–42.

Ralph-Campbell, K., S.L. Pohar, L.M. Guirguis, and E.L. Toth. 2006. "Aboriginal Participation in the DOVE Study." *Canadian Journal of Public Health* 97, no. 4: 305–9.

Reading, C.L., and F. Wien. 2009. *Health Inequalities and Social Determinants of Aboriginal Peoples Health*. Prince George, BC: National Collaborating Centre for Aboriginal Peoples Health.

Riediger, N.D., L.M. Lix, V. Lukianchuk, and S. Bruce. 2014. "Trends in Diabetes and Cardiometabolic Conditions in a Canadian First Nation Community, 2002–2003 to 2011–2012." *Preventing Chronic Disease* 11, no. E198. https://pubmed.ncbi.nlm.nih.gov/25393746/.

Rose, G., F. Duerksen, E. Trepman, M. Cheang, J.N. Simonsen, J. Koulack, H. Fong, et al. 2008. "Multidisciplinary Treatment of Diabetic Foot Ulcers in Canadian Aboriginal and non-Aboriginal People." *Foot Ankle Surgery* 14, no. 2: 74–81.

Shah, B.R., K. Cauch-Dudek, and L. Pigeau. 2011. "Diabetes Prevalence and Care in the Métis Population of Ontario, Canada." *Diabetes Care* 34, no. 12: 2555–56.

Shaw, J.E., R.A. Sicree, and P.Z. Zimmet. 2010. "Global Estimates of the Prevalence of Diabetes for 2010 and 2030." *Diabetes Research and Clinical Practice* 87, no. 1: 4–14.

Statistics Canada. 2006. *Aboriginal Peoples in Canada in 2006: 2006 Census, First Nations People*. Ottawa: Statistics Canada.

Statistics Canada. 2010. *Diabetes, 2010.* Data from the CCHS. http://www.statcan.gc.ca/pub/82-625-x/2011001/article/11459-eng.htm.

Tobe, S., L. Vincent, J. Wentworth, D. Hildebrandt, A. Kiss, N. Perkins, S. Hartman, et al. 2010. "Blood Pressure 2 Years after a Chronic Disease Management Intervention Study." *International Journal of Circumpolar Health* 69, no. 1: 50–60.

Tobe, S.W., G. Pylypchuk, J. Wentworth, A. Kiss, J.P. Szalai, N. Perkins, S. Hartman, et al. 2006. "Effect of Nurse-directed Hypertension Treatment among First Nations People with Existing Hypertension and Diabetes Mellitus: The Diabetes Risk Evaluation and Microalbuminuria (DREAM 3) Randomized Controlled Trial." *Canadian Medical Association Journal* 174, no. 9: 1267–71.

Waldram, J., D.A. Herring, and T.K. Young. 2006. *Aboriginal Health in Canada: Historical, Cultural and Epidemiological Perspectives 2nd Edition.* Toronto: University of Toronto Press.

Whiting, D., N. Unwinm, and G. Roglic. 2010. "Diabetes: Equity and Social Determinants." In *Equity, Social Determinants and Public Health Programmes*, edited by E. Blas and A.S. Kurup, 77–94. Geneva, Switzerland: World Health Organization. http://whqlibdoc. who.int/publications/2010/9789241563970_eng.pdf.

Willows, N.D. 2005. "Determinants of Healthy Eating in Aboriginal Peoples in Canada: The Current State of Knowledge and Research Gaps." *Canadian Journal of Public Health* 96, Supplement 3: S32–36.

Young, T.K., J. Reading, B. Elias, and J.D. O'Neil. 2000. "Type 2 Diabetes Mellitus in Canada's First Nations: Status of an Epidemic in Progress." *Canadian Medical Association Journal* 163, no. 5: 561–66.

Yu, C.H., and B. Zinman. 2007. "Type 2 Diabetes and Impaired Glucose Tolerance in Aboriginal Populations: A Global Perspective." *Diabetes Research and Clinical Practice* 78, no. 2: 159–70.

12   *"Here," "Now," and Health Research*

Developing Shared Priorities within Scholarship

GINETTA SALVALAGGIO

Ginetta Salvalaggio is a family physician who works with urban underserved patients in Edmonton, many of whom are Indigenous Peoples. This chapter was developed from her oral presentation at the Wisdom Engaged: Traditional Knowledge for Northern Community Well-Being conference, which took place in Edmonton, Alberta, in February 2015. Dr. Salvalaggio speaks to important issues on how physicians and medical researchers can work with urban underserved community members in a respectful collaboration to address the substantial health issues faced by this community. The reader is introduced to a spectrum of approaches to health research to show how the outcomes of research are shaped by the methods chosen, and what the strengths and weaknesses of each are.

Introduction

Many northern people have ties to both their home communities and distant urban areas.[1] This mobility leads to new relationships in adopted communities, with the unique composition, culture, and priorities of urban Indigenous communities facing change on a constant basis. Clinicians, researchers, and urban Indigenous communities wishing to engage with each other do not have a pre-existing road map, and may find themselves learning protocols for local engagement in real time. The "here" and "now" immediacy inherent in the knowledge and action needs of evolving communities needs to be balanced with a commitment to sound scholarship and partnership. Four traditions provide complementary ways of knowing and advocacy approaches from which partners in health research can draw wisdom and balance:

1. *Conventional scientific inquiry* generates verifiable, empirical data from measurable phenomena.
2. *Knowledge translation* collates, synthesizes, and adapts existing knowledge for use in real-world settings by a variety of stakeholders.
3. *Participatory action research* creates community-led knowledge that is community-relevant and actionable.
4. *Harm reduction* promotes community well-being through innovation and advocacy.

Urban Landscapes as Traditional Gathering Places

Throughout history, humans have been social beings, relying on functional family and community units to thrive. These communities have not existed in isolation, instead interacting with one another for mutual benefit to trade, to share knowledge, and sometimes to join together. Turtle Island's peoples are no exception to this human intermingling, identifying natural gathering places to which they have regularly returned for centuries. Although over time the drivers and nature of human gatherings have changed, often the gathering places remain the same—prime trading locations with plentiful resources. In many cases, pre-colonization gathering places have become today's post-colonization cities—permanent urban settings influenced by Indigenous Nations and settlers alike (Carli 2013).

Redefining Community

Urban Indigenous communities glean their membership from multiple existing communities across Turtle Island (INAC 1996). Community members vary in their length of urban residence and intention to stay. Maintaining one's Indigenous cultural identity in an urban minority environment comes with unique challenges (INAC 1996; Carli 2013). For example, who is the face of a community in flux? Who speaks for a community in constant transition? This membership and leadership plasticity creates a culture of immediacy—although lived experience informs it, the community also defines itself and determines its priorities according to who is here, now.

Finding Balance and Drawing Wisdom from Each Other

Communities experiencing constant change present unique considerations for successful academic–urban Indigenous partnerships. Engaged researchers may discover a tremendous amount of passion, innovation, and pragmatism among community members, along with a commitment to sharing knowledge that will help the community as quickly and openly as possible. Participants in community–academic gatherings include regular faces over time but also others who come and go. Community leaders and spokespersons are not necessarily Elders or Chiefs. Several Nations participate, and as such, meetings can vary considerably from traditional, non-urban Protocol.

Urban scholars, then, balance older and newer ways of knowing in their work. Scientifically sound research and traditional academic definitions of success may at first seem in tension with current standards for knowledge translation and community engagement, particularly when the research setting involves a rapidly evolving community. However, these wisdom traditions integrate well when they are understood and valued by all project parties. Further, a relatively new grassroots movement with urban origins—harm reduction—provides an additional lens from which to engage in urban research in a culturally aware manner. The balance of this chapter will review the history, approach, benefits, and risks of these four wisdom traditions, and explore how these traditions can work together equitably to improve the health and well-being of urban communities.

I will explore these themes through a fictional case study that was created to help illustrate common interactions between the wisdom traditions. Any resemblance to real people, groups, or places is not intentional.

Vignette: A Community Identifies an Emerging Concern

About five thousand Indigenous people currently reside in a midsize Canadian city. Many of the community's youth attend the same high school. In the past six months, a dozen students have been hospitalized or died due to drug poisoning. The community is reeling with this development and wants to act quickly to prevent further drug poisoning from happening. Mâmawi (Together), an advocacy group of local Indigenous women, reaches out to Jan, a researcher at the local university, who has worked with the group before.

Wisdom Tradition 1: Scientific Inquiry

History

Humans have universally observed and experimented with their environment since before recorded history, synthesizing acquired experiences into knowledge to be transmitted to later generations. Over time, an empirical approach to knowledge acquisition, emphasizing objectivity and reason, gained increasing prominence in the European world view. Aristotle articulated a systematic approach to scientific inquiry that the Renaissance later embraced and conventional scientists have continued to refine to the present day (Gotthelf 2012; Woodcock 2014).

Approach

As science has diversified, specific sequences used to generate new knowledge vary considerably for each discipline (Woodcock 2014). Typically, however, scientists adhere to several core methodological tenets; health scientists are no exception. First, observation precedes experimentation. Scientists either observe phenomena themselves, or learn of phenomena observed by others. These observations form the basis for hypothesis generation. Scientists then design an experiment to test their hypothesis, carry out the experiment, and obtain the data needed to confirm or refute their hypothesis. Minimization of potential bias, systematic adherence to experimental protocol, and rigorous documentation of observations and experimental steps help scientists to ensure their studies are reproducible and their results are valid. Methods and results are reported, traditionally to other scientists, to contribute to the existing body of knowledge and encourage the generation of new hypotheses.

Science does not exist in a vacuum, and several ancillary activities co-occur with the core tenets of inquiry. Hypotheses are frequently refined with additional consultation and literature review. Experiments require financial and infrastructure resources to be carried out, and as such, most modern scientists receive formal support from academic institutions, government, industry, and other funding bodies. Ethics boards review studies and provide approval prior to the beginning of experimentation. Scientists then hire staff and mentor students as part of the study. These study teams generate manuscripts, presentations, and other traditional forms of dissemination of study results. Scientific peers review grant applications, abstracts, and manuscripts to ensure they are methodologically sound and worthy of funding and/or dissemination.

Benefits

Provided these steps are followed, conventional scientific research can provide powerful and relevant health sciences knowledge to communities. Valid results generated in one setting can potentially be reproduced in and generalized to other settings. Scientific knowledge can support or refute existing standards of care, thus encouraging evidence-based practice. Newly tested tools can be adopted in practice to improve health care provision and subsequent health outcomes. Health service funders can justify investing in evidence-based interventions, and communities and health care providers can justify engaging in controversial but evidence-based work.

Risks

When scientists and their conventional support structures adopt an insular approach to knowledge generation, scientific inquiry is capable of minimal impact at best and great harm at worst. The possibility of return on investment can afford disproportionate power to investors, and may dictate which studies get funded and which never see the light of day. Overreliance on external stakeholder priorities and/or observations, and under-reliance on patient and community experience, may lead scientists to generate irrelevant and inappropriate hypotheses. Assuming scientists ask the right question, minimal or absent community consultation can lead to invalid or unfeasible study design and inaccurate interpretation, with the wrong answer obtained as a result. Worse yet, a colonialist approach to data collection sacrifices ethical conduct in research for the sake of adherence to methodology and scientist advancement.

Even when the above pitfalls are avoided, research can take a long time, and findings can be potentially hard to decipher. Communities in which research takes place may struggle to understand why priority answers are not forthcoming more quickly. Traditionally, few researchers have received training in effective communication of their findings and overemphasize technical language and academic dissemination venues. Poor research communication promotes poor research uptake.

A response to suboptimal research uptake is the evidence-based medicine (EBM) movement (Evidence Based Medicine Working Group 1992). Inundated with an ocean of research noise, clinician consumers of knowledge critically appraise available research findings according to relevance, validity, importance, and applicability to practice. In keeping with conventional scientific methodology, practitioners assign greater worth to prospective, randomized, blinded, controlled interventional studies at low risk of bias, particularly large studies with greater statistical power. The perceived strength of these studies promotes their uptake into practice. In contrast, observational, retrospective, and small-scale exploratory research, whether qualitative or quantitative, is perceived as weak evidence and systematically undervalued. Taken to the extreme, the positivist epistemology currently dominating health sciences discourse construes hypothesis-supported theory as absolute truth, and leaves little to no room for the art of medicine and alternative ways of knowing.

Vignette: A Partnering Scholar Uses Scientific Inquiry
to Help Address the Concern
Jan expected to hear from Mâmawi, as the media have reported extensively on the recent drug poisoning events. She agrees to meet, and begins to prepare notes. Jan obtains public health bulletins outlining the results of toxicology

testing for the first few cases, and conducts a preliminary literature review on drug poisoning prevention interventions. She consults with analyst colleagues affiliated with the regional health authority to determine what administrative health data are available to measure the impact of any interventions.

Wisdom Tradition 2: Knowledge Translation

History

The advent of the EBM (evidence-based medicine) movement has certainly benefitted the health sciences, in that it has challenged the research community to consider the implications of research findings for the consumers of that knowledge. However, audiences cannot critically appraise and assign relative value to research findings if researchers fail to make their findings accessible. Further, the digital age bombards clinicians daily with new information and new formats; sense making is an increasingly complex task. The field of knowledge translation (KT)—evidence-based medicine is a domain therein— has evolved over the past half-century in response to this evidence-to-practice gap (Estabrooks et al. 2008). Its current prominence is such that major research funding bodies mandate an a priori comprehensive knowledge translation plan, and academic institutions are gradually recognizing research impact via nonscientific dissemination venues.

Approach

Knowledge translation is, at its heart, a science of communication. KT specialists connote the scope of this field through the frequent use of several related words—"transfer," "synthesis," "exchange," "sharing," "utilization," "mobilization," "implementation." The knowledge-to-action cycle (Figure 12.1) captures the cyclical nature of knowledge tailoring and adaptation for real-world settings (Graham et al. 2006). Unlike traditional end-of-project strategies for scientific dissemination, comprehensive knowledge translation is iterative, occurring and recurring at several points throughout the process of knowledge generation. Effective KT tends to be active as opposed to passive, multipronged, relevant to local needs, and informed by multiple stakeholders (Straus, Tetroe, and Graham 2009). Ideally, researchers allocate sufficient

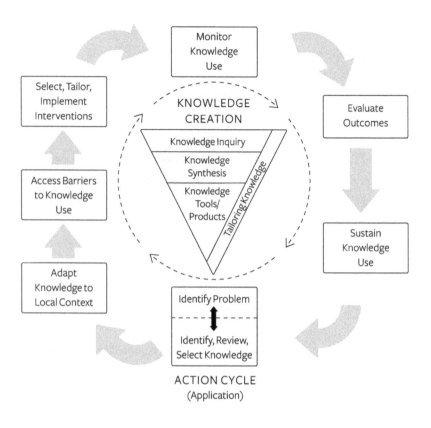

FIGURE 12.1 *Knowledge-to-Action Cycle (Graham 2006, 19).*

resources within their labs to sustain their KT efforts over time, and evaluate the impact of these knowledge translation efforts.

The context in which knowledge translation takes place depends on the messenger, the message, and the audience. Plain language summaries uploaded to a social media platform, point-of-care decision support tools embedded in an electronic medical record, and community sharing circles are examples of potential evidence-based communication strategies, but will not have universal impact for all knowledge or all users of knowledge.

Benefits

Knowledge needs to be shared to be meaningful. Knowledge translation creates meaning out of scientific inquiry; it takes research and makes it adaptive and accessible. It provides a standardized framework for interacting with knowledge, including understanding a community's knowledge needs, knowing where to find and how to interpret knowledge relevant to those needs, sharing this knowledge in the right way with the right people, and evaluating whether this communication is effective.

Risks

Assuming that the knowledge a given community needs exists to begin with, and researchers ensure it is accessible, inadequate subsequent attention to all aspects of the knowledge-to-action cycle can nevertheless produce ineffective KT results. Knowledge translation strategies commonly in use today emphasize knowledge tailoring and are gradually increasing emphasis on addressing barriers to knowledge uptake, monitoring knowledge use, and evaluation. Unfortunately, two time- and resource-intensive components of the cycle—adaptation to local context and sustained knowledge use—are cursorily addressed by under-resourced teams. For example, an academic team might characterize an externally created online survey as a sufficient stakeholder needs assessment, but the stakeholder map might be incomplete, some stakeholders might not be able to read or have access to the internet, and the survey questions might have nothing to do with stakeholder priorities. Another team might enjoy tremendous early success getting the word out about its findings and report a change in practice as a result of its KT strategy, but subsequently lose the energy behind its knowledge translation efforts with the end of project funding and learn that knowledge users have not sustained the practice change on their own.

Unfortunately, although KT does not imply unidirectional transfer of knowledge, the health sciences culture tends to interpret knowledge translation in this way. Health professionals, physicians in particular, have classically viewed themselves (and been viewed by the public) as authoritative purveyors of healing and knowledge for people in need. The inherent power differential in this classical view, however benevolent it might be, encourages a quasi-colonial pushing out of knowledge without any pulling in. KT practitioners mindful of this tendency will favour terminology such as "knowledge exchange" and "knowledge sharing" to convey the importance of bidirectional communication.

Vignette: Partners Synthesize and Share Available Scientific and Community Knowledge

Jan's graduate student, Marc, is interested in mental health issues. Jan asks Marc to compile the results of their literature review on drug poisoning prevention interventions. Although enhanced depression case finding, community-based naloxone distribution, and school-based awareness programs are interventions that have some documented evidence of effectiveness with similar study populations, it's not yet clear whether any of these would be acceptable or feasible in their setting. Marc prepares a plain language summary of the literature review, and with guidance from Jan, develops some preliminary questions for possible use in community consultation.

Wisdom Tradition 3: Participatory Action Research
History

Though the concept of scientific inquiry as a means to solve real-world problems in meaningful collaboration with stakeholders can be traced as far back as Aristotle, the subsequent millennia and prevailing sociopolitical forces have largely subordinated the pragmatic and community-driven in favour of the theoretical and tightly controlled (Elliott 2011). The rise of emancipation, Marxism, and anti-colonialism over the last century created the right conditions for science to re-explore its democratic roots (Elliott 2011). It is no longer ethically acceptable to engage in scientific inquiry in a community setting without involving the community as much as possible throughout project design, data collection, interpretation, and dissemination (INAC 1996; Government of Canada 2018). Researchers now have access to clearly articulated guiding principles for meaningful community participation when deciding to engage in community-based scholarship (Allen et al. 2017).

Approach

Participatory action research (PAR) recognizes that knowledge needs to be relevant and helpful to the community seeking it, and that this knowledge can come from unconventional sources. The community co-owns the process of knowledge creation and sharing with researchers. PAR does not restrict itself to a single epistemology, and instead embraces whatever methodological approach is appropriate to knowledge needs. The extent to which the community is an equal partner follows a continuum; community-academic collaborations usually require several years to mature. Typically, researchers will initially reach out to a community by requesting to consult with them on upcoming scholarly work; communities may offer guidance, or alternately decline to participate. In more developed relationships, the community may be the one to reach out to researchers with a question. Researchers ideally limit their role to providing methodological expertise and wrap-around supports (ethics submissions, grant applications, data management, etc.) as requested, whereas the community determines ideal project design, timelines, and dissemination. Researchers may or may not act as data managers, custodians, and co-authors for data owned by the community from which they were derived; these roles can vary and are jointly established by both parties.

Benefits

Researchers choosing to engage in PAR reduce the cultural risks associated with conventional scientific inquiry and knowledge translation (Allen et al. 2017). Rather than acting as the passive source of data and recipient of unidirectional, externally controlled evidence, the community becomes an active and equal participant in scientific inquiry and bidirectional KT. PAR embraces multiple ways of knowing, and affords relevance, validity, and credibility to community-acquired research data (Jagosh et al. 2012, 319–23). Researchers in a long-term community partnership can more easily conduct scholarly work within a community, and communities can more readily access research expertise (Jagosh et al. 2012). Participatory action research contributes to community capacity building and can facilitate sociopolitical change (Jagosh et al. 2012).

Risks

PAR addresses many shortcomings associated with conventional scientific inquiry and knowledge translation, but introduces new challenges to the research process. Researchers and communities need to jointly set a priori expectations, from appropriate protocol for community meetings, to the delegation of responsibility for data collection and dissemination, to the establishment of conflict resolution procedures (Allen et al. 2017). If collaborators have inconsistent expectations of the partnership, their ability to manage conflict arising from unanticipated research findings, dissemination planning, or breaches in research protocol may have serious consequences for both the academic's research program and the community's well-being.

Entering into a PAR relationship requires an investment in time and a willingness to adapt research methods to a community's needs. Unless researchers explicitly factor the establishment of shared community-academic research goals into their research timelines, external stakeholders such as funders and academic institutions may perceive potential associated threats to research protocol fidelity and achievement of project milestones.

Vignette: The Community Leads a Meeting between Partners
in Preparation for Joint Scholarship

Mâmawi members prepare a meal for their meeting with Jan and Marc. Two local Elders, Tom and Yvonne, will attend and lead the group in a smudge and opening prayer. Many of Mâmawi's members have children enrolled in the affected school, and they invite the high school principal, a mental health worker, the public health nurse assigned to the school, and some of the senior students to join the gathering. Mâmawi chooses a long-time member, Annie, to coordinate the project. Annie has a special interest in youth issues and is excited to get more involved in research.

History

The modern harm reduction movement finds its roots in the public health response to the AIDS epidemic of the 1980s (Collins et al. 2012). European, North American, and Australian health care providers observed sharp increases in morbidity and mortality among people who inject drugs, and conventional abstinence-oriented and enforcement-heavy approaches were failing to curb this reality. Beyond AIDS, the dominant drug policy discourses of the period exposed people who use drugs to poverty, incarceration, violence, stigmatization, and other profound threats to well-being (Collins et al. 2012, 10–20). As a result, what began as a public health crisis response specific to the harms associated with drug injection has evolved into a primarily grassroots-driven, humanistic movement for socially marginalized urban populations in general.

Approach

Like scientific inquiry, harm reduction relies on extensive observation. The response to observation, however, is drastically different. People at risk of harm, in partnership with front-line nurses, social workers, and outreach workers, develop innovative and practical ways to reduce risk. Access to these solutions is intentionally low threshold and value neutral (Collins et al. 2012), and innovations are commonly low cost. Examples of harm reduction innovation include sterile needle and syringe provision, drug poisoning response training, and managed alcohol programming.

Harm reduction interventions develop at a meteoric rate; early implementation frequently occurs prior to any conclusive scientific evidence of effectiveness. However, this should not imply that harm reduction practitioners and communities dismiss the value of scholarship. Epidemiologic information, both formal and anecdotal, is constantly shared to identify new approaches to problematic trends. If early success is observed with a new intervention, harm reductionists want to document and celebrate this success widely, and will partner with academics to capture their success and get the word out. Communities organize themselves to passionately and adeptly advocate for any measures that stand to benefit their collective health (Carter and MacPherson 2013; Jürgens 2005).

Benefits

Like PAR, harm reduction emphasizes the meaningful participation of communities in solving problems affecting their health. Harm reduction interventions frequently develop from the grassroots up, lending tremendous community credibility to these approaches. Researchers engaging with harm reduction-oriented communities can more readily include extremely hard to reach individuals in the research process, and can provide substantial support for community capacity-building efforts—including acting as a vehicle for community advocacy.

Harm reductionists understand that knowledge can save lives, and that it needs to be shared in a timely fashion. There is a palpable immediacy and accessibility to the KT of harm reduction; harm reduction scholarship is highly unlikely to gather dust on an academic's bookshelf.

Risks

The very immediacy that lends passion and credibility to the harm reduction movement turns the notion of traditional scientific inquiry on its head. Implementing a harm reduction intervention with high potential benefit holds much higher priority than testing its effectiveness beforehand. Researchers become involved to document effectiveness, however, study design is necessarily pragmatic and at risk of systematic bias as a result. Ethics approval to formally study an intervention may need to be sought after the intervention is already occurring. Further, though harm reductionists are highly skilled advocates and communicators, they may require assistance in communicating their message (and gathering meaningful data) for certain audiences, such as prospective funders and health service providers. Community leaders and messengers may change at a relatively rapid rate as individuals move in and out of the community due to family, work, or health issues. The time-intensive, future-oriented nature of conventional scholarship may frustrate a dynamic community oriented primarily to its present reality.

Vignette: Directly Affected Community Members Contribute Their Expertise
Jay and Amanda are two high school seniors who agree to attend the meeting.
Both have witnessed drug poisoning events among their peers and called for
help when it happened. They wish they had first aid training to help until
professionals arrived. They are also shaken up by what has happened and
have informally started a peer support group for drug poisoning survivors and
witnesses. They need more resources and mentorship to keep it going.

Learning from Each Other

Integrating the wisdom traditions of scientific inquiry, knowledge translation, participatory action research, and harm reduction stands to benefit
all stakeholders in urban Indigenous health research by generating highly
relevant, credible, accessible, and actionable knowledge. Successful integration is contingent on a commitment by all parties to enter into meaningful
relationship with each other. Each tradition has a protocol and a history
(Table 12.1). Research partners may hold expertise in one protocol, but should
have a working knowledge of the other protocols, and be willing to adapt to
meet the collective needs of the partnership.

*Vignette: Partners Draw on Multiple Traditions to Address
Community Concerns*
The first group meeting takes place on an evening, two weeks after it is called,
in the common room of the local friendship centre. Annie introduces the
Elders and, after Ceremony, all around the circle are invited to speak in turn
about their perspective on the recent events, what they would like to see
happen, and how they would like to help. Marc and Annie offer to take notes
of the discussion.

The group reaches consensus that a combination of school-based awareness and drug poisoning response training interventions could be adapted to
meet the needs of Jay, Amanda, and other students in their peer support work.
All agree that traditional Indigenous teachings must be included in order to
promote student and community healing; Tom and Yvonne offer to provide
the student group with this guidance. The school administrator, counsellor, and

nurse commit to allocating space and infrastructure, communicating with other staff and parents, as well as teaching students mental health first aid, basic life support, and naloxone administration. Mâmawi will organize a community awareness campaign and act as the community liaison for the project.

After reviewing notes from the first meeting, Mâmawi and Jan co-develop three research questions: (1) What are the perceived causes of youth drug poisonings? (2) How do youth drug poisonings affect the community? and (3) What is the impact of the local intervention on drug poisoning rates and community well-being? They will adopt a mixed methods design to answer these questions, using student and broader community sharing circles and complemented by available epidemiologic data. Annie and Marc prepare an ethics submission and focus group interview guides together. Jan identifies possible funding sources and applies for a grant to support research costs such as transcription, software, and Marc and Annie's hours on the project.

Jay and Amanda get the word out on social media about their support group and upcoming training and wellness activities. Many new students join the group and learn how to help when someone is at risk of a poisoning event or experiencing one. Tom and Yvonne take interested students on a weekend camping trip and lead them in recreation and other healing activities. Annie and Marc co-moderate sharing circles that are occurring concurrently for the research project, and perform qualitative analyses with guidance from Jan. Jan obtains drug poisoning data from the health authority for the periods prior to and after the launch of enhanced student support group activities.

Mâmawi convenes the original stakeholder group to discuss research results and assist Annie, Marc, and Jan with the interpretation of findings. All are excited to see proof that their collaboration is helping to meet youth needs and reduce drug poisoning rates. Some community members in attendance disclose how emotionally difficult the work can be, and how occasionally personal safety is at risk with this work. Mâmawi and Jan commit to exploring how the risks associated with the intervention can be addressed.

Mâmawi shares the study results at a few local gatherings with residents, and also via its social media accounts and through the free community newspaper, which is widely read by residents. Jan has communications support at the university and requests help to prepare a plain language summary for online distribution to health sector stakeholders. Jan, Annie, and Marc also begin work on a scientific manuscript, and prepare an oral presentation for an upcoming mental health conference. Annie ensures other Mâmawi members have the opportunity to provide input on all written and oral material prior to release, and participates as a presenter at the conference. Mâmawi, Jay, and Amanda want to champion this project locally and ask Jan to identify key health sector leaders who may be interested in co-championing their cause.

Conclusion

Academic partnerships with urban Indigenous communities can be successful, provided team members apply the best that each wisdom tradition has to offer for any given scholarship situation. Team members must equally anticipate potential pitfalls and jointly create a plan to deal with them should they occur. The "here" and "now" energy of urban Indigenous communities is well suited to the passion of the harm reduction approach; balanced with a commitment to scientific rigour, comprehensive knowledge sharing, and relationship building, health research within urban Indigenous communities can be tremendously powerful and rewarding for all partners.

TABLE 12.1 *A Comparison of Wisdom Traditions through the Research Trajectory*

	Scientific Inquiry	Knowledge Translation	Action Research	Harm Reduction
QUESTION	Derived from literature review, observation, and identified knowledge gaps	Takes into account several stakeholders and local context; draws on existing evidence	Asked by community; relevant to local needs	Driven by local trends and needs; action often needed quickly
DESIGN	Mitigation of bias; measurement accuracy; comparability	Based on knowledge-to-action cycle	Specific approach shaped and approved by community; culturally aware	Practical, low-cost, innovative; originates in community
IMPLEMENTATION	Coordinated; adherence to protocol	Coordinated, pre-planned; adapted to local context	Coordinated, in partnership with community	Comparatively quick, involving front line and community
EVALUATION	Traditionally quantitative; pre-planned	Quantitative and qualitative; pre-planned	Quantitative and qualitative; pre-planned but may evolve	Quantitative and qualitative; may develop in tandem with project
DISSEMINATION	Publication; academic presentations	Scientific; policy; clinical; public	Driven by community, owned by community	Informal first, more formal later

NOTE

1. This chapter is dedicated to the Indigenous members of Edmonton's urban underserved community, who continue to teach me every day about what it means to be a settler-ally. I offer this account in the spirit of reconciliation.

REFERENCES

Allen, M.L., J. Salsberg, M. Knot, J.W. LeMaster, M. Felzien, J.M. Westfall, C.P. Herbert, et al. 2017. "Engaging with Communities, Engaging with Patients: Amendment to the NAPCRG 1998 Policy Statement on Responsible Research with Communities." *Family Practice* 34, no. 3: 313–21.

Carli, V. 2013. "The City as a 'Space of Opportunity': Urban Indigenous Experiences and Community Safety Partnerships." In *Well-Being in the Urban Aboriginal Community*, edited by D. Newhouse, K. FitzMaurice, T. McGuire-Adams, and D. Jetté, 1–21. Toronto: Thompson Educational Publishing.

Carter, C.I., and D. MacPherson. 2013. *Getting to Tomorrow: A Report on Canadian Drug Policy*. Burnaby, BC: Canadian Drug Policy Coalition, Simon Fraser University

Collins, S.E., L. Seema, D.E. Logan Slifasefi, L.S. Samples, J.M. Somers, and G.A. Marlatt. 2012. "Current Status, Historical Highlights, and Basic Principles of Harm Reduction." In *Harm Reduction: Pragmatic Strategies for Managing High Risk Behaviors*, edited by G.A. Marlatt, M.E. Larimer, and K. Witkiewitz, 3–35. New York: Guilford.

Elliott, P.W. 2011. *Participatory Action Research: Challenges, Complications, and Opportunities*. Saskatoon: Centre for the Study of Co-operatives, University of Saskatchewan.

Estabrooks, C.A., L. Derksen, C. Winther, J.N. Lavis, S.D. Scott, L. Wallin, J. Profetto-McGrath. 2008. "The Intellectual Structure and Substance of the Knowledge Utilization Field: A Longitudinal Author Co-Citation Analysis." *BMC Implementation Science* 3, no. 49: 1–22.

Evidence-Based Medicine Working Group. 1992. "Evidence-Based Medicine: A New Approach to Teaching the Practice of Medicine." *Journal of the American Medical Association* 268, no. 17: 2420–25.

Gotthelf, A. 2012. *Teleology, First Principles, and Scientific Method in Aristotle's Biology*. Oxford: Oxford University Press.

Government of Canada. 2018. "TCPS 2—Chapter 9: Research Involving the First Nations, Inuit and Métis Peoples of Canada." https://ethics.gc.ca/eng/tcps2-eptc2_2018_chapter9-chapitre9.html.

Graham, I.D., J. Logan, M.B. Harrison, S.E. Straus, J. Tetroe, W. Caswell, and N. Robertson. 2006. "Lost in Knowledge Translation: Time for a Map?" *Journal of Continuing Education in the Health Professions* 26, no. 1: 13–24.

Indian and Northern Affairs Canada (INAC). 1996. *Report of the Royal Commission on Aboriginal Peoples.* https://www.bac-lac.gc.ca/eng/discover/aboriginal-heritage/royal-commission-aboriginal-peoples/Pages/final-report.aspx.

Jagosh, J., A.C. Macaulay, P. Pluye, J. Salsberg, P.L. Bush, J. Henderson, E. Sirett, et al. 2012. "Uncovering the Benefits of Participatory Research: Implications of a Realist Review for Health Research and Practice." *Millbank Quarterly* 90, no. 2: 311–46.

Jürgens, R. 2005. *"Nothing about us without us": Greater, Meaningful Involvement of People Who Use Illegal Drugs: A Public Health, Ethical, and Human Rights Imperative.* Toronto: Canadian HIV/AIDS Legal Network.

Straus, S., J. Tetroe, and I.D. Graham. 2009. *Knowledge Translation in Health Care: Moving from Evidence to Practice.* Hoboken, NJ: Wiley-Blackwell.

Woodcock, B.A. 2014. "'The Scientific Method' as Myth and Ideal." *Science and Education* 23: 2069–93.

13   *Nature Is Medicine*

ALLISON KELLIHER

*Allison Kelliher is a Traditional Healer descended from a family with
healing gifts, and is the first Koyukon Athabascan medical doctor. Formerly
with Southcentral Foundation, she is the only physician formally trained and
certified as a Tribal Doctor, and is now faculty at the University of North
Dakota and maintains a private practice in Alaska. Her goal is to empower
Indigenous voice in medicine and improve access to traditional modalities.
This chapter relies on countless experiences and dialogue with healers
over years.*

Introduction

It is a great honour to be gifted with an opportunity to share and give back
to the community through writing about nature as medicine. I write with
gratitude and respect for the teachings that I carry. My teachers say that, as
Traditional Healers, we are vessels for knowledge and healing, conduits of
energy that comes from the Creator. The work we do takes into account all
parts of being: body, mind, emotions, and energy or spirit. Our hope is that
each and every community is inspired to support the tradition of healers.

Traditional Indigenous medicines offer effective treatment for chronic
disease prevention and treatment. The burden of chronic disease is largely

influenced by our modern lifestyle. Our traditional ways offer insight and opportunity for healthier lifeways to be remembered and practised again. Three main elements of air, water, and earth are described here from the Traditional Healing perspective. These elements can be used for healing in ways that are not limited to those ways listed.

Mainstream (Western) health care limits standard treatment options such that it often excludes modalities that may help and pose less risk for harm. Too often, these options include powerful pharmaceuticals, traumatic procedures, and referrals that take time and resources. Many of these options fall short of treatment goals, and place the patient at risk for side effects. There is a dire need today for different treatment strategies that patients find more helpful, including options that carry a low risk of harm, those that improve quality of life, and those that contribute to overall wellness. Ancient ethnomedicines and Traditional Healing treatments have existed for as long as we can recall, and are increasingly being tested and proven to benefit. In time, our ways will be recognized as valuable, and will have a place in helping to heal ourselves and provide resources for others to restore balance. Our ways promote harmony by paying attention to the delicate sacred nature of the interconnected universe.

My goal, as a family and integrative physician, and as an Alaska Native Traditional Healer, is to promote natural ways of healing and foster under-standing in order to blend the best of Western medicine with the other healing systems. Further, contributing to the body of knowledge in accepted science, and facilitating opportunity for students and scholars to access and practise and appreciate our ways, would be of benefit.

Sharing Story

Alaska Native People have always shared stories. Our oral history and connection to the land are what we value and have passed down for generations. Story is at the centre of our culture, daily life, and traditional education. Traditional teachings are often subtle, recur, and are experiential. I share some of my story so you know the perspective I speak from, and to encourage others to continue their healing journey and have a frame of reference when pursuing health and healing.

My parents remember the time I was born as one of the coldest on the coast of the Bering Sea. It was the year of the photo finish on the Iditarod race, a race that commemorated triumph over disease utilizing traditional technology: the dog sled. I was named after my maternal grandmother, Alice Hildebrand, from the Middle Yukon, Dine, or Koyukon Athabaskan people of Nulato and follow her Clan line. We are the Middle of the River Clan, who represent resiliency in the great king salmon who continue to guide my work. My middle name is shared with my Auntie Miranda Wright, anthropologist, leader, and culture bearer. My Aunties provide a wonderful gift of knowledge, strength, support, and inspiration. My father's people emigrated from beautiful County Kerry, Ireland, due to social unrest. When I was a child, after receiving my vaccines at the local clinic, I was gifted my traditional name Kasgnoc, from Katherine, whose husband from King Island had just passed. I knew from a young age that I could see, hear, and feel things that others might not. I was trained from a young age in the arts of hands-on healing and plant medicine. The path to becoming a Medicine Person is determined by the community who names us as such, and I am honoured for the support of my ancestors and teachers who allow me to share these things.

My family became my original teachers. Caring, capable people surrounded me with such rich heritage I continue to discover more about. Grandma Alice Hildebrand taught my mother to "walk in both worlds," to respect the old and traditional ways that had sustained our people for so long, and to accept the technological advances and cultural change that were upon us. My Mother, Trudy "Dumplings" Kelliher, was able to succeed in the modern world and practise the old ways, thanks to, and despite, her experience in boarding school. She was able to instill in us intimacy with, and reverence for, the land, allowing access to something greater than us. Her capability as a caretaker, bead worker, seamstress, small and large game hunter, expert fish cutter, impeccable fire keeper, and gold miner continues to amaze me. I remember her teachings daily: to foster love for ourselves so that we can share love with others; she said if you didn't love yourself first, you couldn't fully love another. We frequently have Elders at our home, pick berries for others, and generally support our community in any way we can. A few of her other teachings are to never be wasteful; always treat things with respect; to try our hardest and be satisfied with the result; to give open-heartedly, show gratitude, be respectful and patient; and that there is no excuse to be bored. She cared for children and animals of all ages. She and her sisters recall raising many wild birds and an orphaned black bear. It wasn't unusual to have at least one extra child living at our home at any given time. She raised us to understand medicine was in our family and was inherited. My Great-Grandmother Agnes had been a Medicine Person, marked as such with a circle tattoo on her hand, and the medicine was to be passed down.

I am often reminded of the importance of the balance of opposites, such as masculine and feminine. I was blessed to have a caring, generous father, Patrick Brendan Kelliher. He and I were born and raised in western Alaska's tiny city of Nome. He taught me many things, such as the value of an education, which he referred to as a "piece of paper." His family had emigrated from Ireland and earned their life off the land and justice. My Grandfather Maurice was a lay judge, advocating for Indigenous perspective after Alaska's statehood. He taught me of humility and commitment to community. One day, we were enjoying fall near Salmon Lake, noting the crimson of what seemed endless spawning red salmon. Father explained lovingly that these parents were giving their life for their children. Recalling this lesson of selflessness, I am still moved to tears. The miracle of salmon is something I took for granted as a child. The salmon are becoming ill from the effects of the extractive economy, reminding us that balance must be restored with practising our traditional ways.

As time went on, I prayed for a teacher, and in time teachers came to me and offered teachings. Some teachings are too sacred to be shared in text, and many teachings are meant to be passed down one on one. When I graduated with my undergraduate degree, I was most honoured to receive a mature eagle feather beaded with a traditional calendar. I would later learn from Terry Maresca, MD, that eagle feathers symbolize the balance of feminine and masculine energies, which I consider similar to the powers of creation and destruction. It is an honour that Tribal Doctor Rita Blumenstein, member of the Council of Indigenous Grandmothers, allowed me to apprentice with her for years. She said, "Go to the east. Bring our medicine back. We sent it to the east during the wars." She explained many of our young people served in these wars, and that our medicine had been sent there. I immediately remembered a song I had known since my first traditional Ceremony, commemorating a young man sent off to a war against an unknown country, and knew she spoke the truth. I have come to find in global travels and learning that how people use medicines is more similar than different. My family, village, and Tribe continue to share and rediscover our wealth of healing modalities. We all use elements of air, water, and earth for healing, and many of us find plants, being close to the earth, as the greatest healers.

For decades I have pursued knowledge and teachings from Elders, healers, teachers, and scientists. I am honoured to be the first physician in my Tribe, and have been inspired by many who have influenced my practice. My family tells of a prophecy that was brought from an Oglala Lakota Tribe. They shared that "Medicine of the future would come from the north. Look to the eagles and remember our relatives in the south." I hope to continue to teach and share our ways of healing to help us remember how to restore balance to ourselves and our system of healing.

Traditional Knowledge

Traditional Knowledge is distinct from Western knowledge, where proof is needed and quantified. Traditional Knowledge is trans-generational, can be inherited, and has value. To put this in perspective, modern humans have existed for approximately 150,000 years (Klein 1995). This is plenty of time to create valuable heritage and knowledge for medicine and wellness. We hold vast and deep teachings. Traditional Knowledge can be described as that which we learn passed down from Elders, or through observation, direct experience, dreaming, Vision Quests, stories, deep connection, and relationship (Krohn 2007). Healing knowledge is highly valued, as our life could depend upon it. It is protected and respected. Some practices are closely guarded by Traditional Knowledge bearers, and others feel an urgency to share. Traditional Knowledge is our way of knowing the world around us and has true value. Healing is a holistic experience that includes the individual transitioning from a state of illness to balance through transformation.

Sometimes Traditional Knowledge leaves our communities only to return. My Auntie Ida tells the story about my Grandfather Eddie Hildebrand teaching schoolchildren and their teacher how to butcher the magnificent, life-giving moose the traditional way, with a pocketknife. Years later, that schoolteacher, having left Nulato, had the opportunity to share this knowledge with a community that had lost all of its teachers of this art, thus allowing the knowledge to return and be practised. For too long these healthful ways have been undervalued. All peoples are indigenous to somewhere, and had healing practices prior to modern medicine. The time is now to revive our wellness practices and work together with others around the globe that are also working toward health and healing and remembering and preserving the traditional ways. We are remembering our right to live healthy naturally.

Traditional Healing honours a connection between spiritual and physical health, just as it has for centuries, and includes a variety of practices. A glimpse at Traditional Healing pre-contact (before 1741) from literature reveals the use of medicinal remedies, surgery, thermal therapy, massage therapy, psychological healing, and spiritual healing. Medicinal remedies utilized plants and animals, administered orally or applied on sites of disease. Surgeries included amputation, bleeding, cautery, dental extraction, removal of arrows and other weapons, bloodletting to allow bad humours to escape, and suturing wounds (Fortuine 1989). Usually, our medicines include a single plant, as they are powerful due to the harsh environment. I have found traditional Ceremonies to be helpful for people, regardless of their cultural background. In my experience, Alaska Native healers generally learn from mentors, who teach and learn through hands-on apprenticeship. Each Traditional Healer is trained uniquely and has an individualized scope of practice and set of skills.

Introduction to the Elements

Maintaining balance in our mind, body, and spirit is fostered by close relationship and complex interactions with the elements. Traditional Alaska Native healers teach the importance of breathing, hydrating, and nourishing our bodies with nature, touch, movement, and nutrition. The following sections divide these concepts into air, water, and earth elements. Built into our traditional lifestyle is the Protocol for harvesting, preparation, and use of each of these medicines, which often entails a great deal of physical activity balancing our originally high fat diets.

Growing up, we knew our responsibility in a remote setting was to care for self, avoiding illness and injury as best we knew how. We enjoyed purpose in our existence and avoided Western treatments at all costs, reserving this for life-threatening situations only. Our wellness, and staying well, was a way of life. A collection of basic practices to promote wellness is found here as a gentle guide to remembering our original instructions.

Air

When we come into the world, one of our first gifts is breath. Through experiences in life, and when we experience pain, our breathing becomes more restricted. Other behaviours, such as smoking, expose our bodies to toxins when the air is not clean. Full, clean, gentle loving breaths and laughter are powerful healing tools that can bring peace of mind. One of our childhood games was *muk*, where we tried to make each other laugh as we quietly distracted each other with silly faces and antics. The first one to laugh lost! I remember this as an early teaching of breath, and how it helps your ability to maintain focus. The breath gives us constant opportunity to practise a calm mind. Additionally, as the breath fills the lungs, the abdominal organs and back muscles are gently massaged. Scents can be added to promote relaxation and healing. My mom remembers that her grandmother used to keep spruce boughs on the back of the stove for health.

One of my favourite practices is focus of the mind to allow us to connect to our bodies by feeling the earth below us, our bodies pressing into the earth, and then allowing the breath to consciously enter through the nose. Some prefer to practise with closed eyes, or by gazing upon a focal point. I encourage whatever is comfortable for you. Gently breathe out through the nose. If you are unable to breathe through your nose, then using your mouth is fine. However, nasal breathe does promote deeper breath through nitric oxide gas stored in the deep nasal passages that serves as a vasodilator and improves oxygen delivery and toxin elimination through the lungs. Gently exhaling completely allows the lungs to fill more easily. Start filling the lungs from the lower portions up to the middle portions into the armpits, and finally into the upper portions at the top of the chest. Then start the cycle over again. Gently exhale from top down, allowing your abdomen to relax on your inhale so your lungs can expand. This simple breathing exercise can help to relieve musculoskeletal tension and dysfunction. Conscious breathing can be a powerful tool to help alleviate neck and back pain, and restore posture and energy for those who tend to be tired or anxious. Breathing is essential for lymphatic flow, which is also essential for immune function.

This type of breath is often referred to as yogic breathing but has also been practised by my Elders for centuries. Studies have confirmed that it helps to balance the autonomic nervous system and is safe for a wide variety of clinical conditions. For example, in those who are survivors of mass disaster and have PTSD, it enhances well-being, mood, attention, focus, and stress tolerance. This type of breathing practice is often combined with yoga postures, other yogic breathing, and meditation. Trained teachers are of benefit when learning these techniques, and at least 20–30 minutes a day is what seems to maximize benefits (Brown and Gerbarg 2005).

Fumigants have been used by our people to cleanse space, and are a powerful way to use breath as medicine. Sage, sweetgrass, cedar, and spruce are used to cleanse, protect, and invite positivity. Aromatherapy is a modern use of plant scent through essential oils used for physical, spiritual, and emotional well-being. I have heard oils referred to as the essence of the plant. I prefer to use oils as aroma, or diluted in oil as a topical application, rather than ingesting these powerful medicines. Topical application must be done carefully as each medicine is unique. There is a need to dilute the concentrated oils, and many benefit pain, inflammation, skin rashes, and infections, although this must be done skillfully, and a knowledgeable teacher is helpful. There are studies that look at the safety and benefits of aromatherapy for treating, or as an adjunct for treatment of, chronic illnesses (see Barati et al. 2016; Brownfield 1998; Buckle 1999; and Itai et al. 2000).

When the brain is quiet and focused in a practiced manner, with steady breath, we call that meditation. Many types of meditation exist. Our Elders and healers used techniques to focus and unite heart and mind for purification and practice. Generally, a heart-centred approach, where focus is on the internal drum, infusing it with love and gratitude is a healthy practice. The idea is to remind the body to feel a sense of harmony at all times to reduce effects of stress and improve our resiliency. It gives your brain time to heal. This practice harmonizes and expands your energy body, of which the heart is a central part. The body is surrounded and penetrated by energy. Modern medicine actually uses these energies when measuring heart and brain tracings. It is not often used as a healing modality in Western medicine, but there are many energy medicine techniques. Healing touch is a particular modality with evidence of benefit (Post-White et al. 2003). Traditional Healing offers a variety of energy medicines, such as in the form of microsystems where the feet and hands are microsystems reflecting the entire body and are stimulated to effect balance and overall health.

Awareness of the importance of breath and how it is central to health will help us to restore balance. I was taught that a calm, open mind in a balanced body allows us to connect to greater sense of belonging and our higher power. If we remember how important cleansing breath is, then perhaps we will learn how to keep it clean and toxify our air less.

Water

Water is essential for life on our planet. Water is often used in healing Ceremony, and has the amazing ability to be liquid, solid, and a gas. Water evaporates off our body throughout the day in our breath. Particular illnesses such as fever and diarrhea can accelerate these losses. Maintaining hydration and using water as medicine can be helpful. One can choose to combine water with medicinal plants as a healing tea. Fasting with water has been used as a powerful medicine. I know of people that have healed from water Ceremony, where water that has been blessed and prayed over intentionally is used as medicine. With guidance from a trusted health care provider, the benefits of fasting can be explored.

Drink clean water throughout the day. This may be more difficult than it sounds initially, as knowing your water is clean can be a challenge. Know your local resources for water and possible contamination. Consider a filtration system, or having your water tested for safety if you are concerned. Many patients have questions about how much water they should drink, and if they are drinking enough water. Each of us is an individual. Thus, knowing your own hydration status and personal needs is best. Ask yourself if you are thirsty, and if you drink water throughout the day. If you are thirsty, and don't drink water throughout the day, you probably need more water. If your urine is dark, this can be a sign of dehydration, and drinking more water can help. Caffeine and other diuretics in teas can lead to relative dehydration. For this and other reasons, I have found that many patients find time away from coffee healthful. If you have trouble waking up at night, needing to go to the bathroom, then avoid drinking water a few hours before bedtime.

Due to potential contaminants in water, I find it helpful to use a water filter and prefer to use filtered water for cooking and drinking. Adequate hydration is necessary for proper elimination of toxins through the kidneys in urine and function of the lubrication of the gut and joints that need turgor to support our weight. Water is essential for all of our bodies' processes and can be a medicine in and of itself.

Earth

When we are raised traditionally, we are in deep relationship with our surroundings, feeling we know the earth like we would our grandmother. Earth medicine includes the importance of our traditional diets, plant medicines, and lifeways, such as body movement, Ceremony, and community that allow us to harvest from an intact ecosystem. Feeling and experiencing physical connection to this element is essential for our people to maintain balance. Body movement and care of our physical body are essential. We are in balance when we are in community. Additionally, earth medicine includes aspects of nutrition and plant medicine. Earth medicine includes caring for the body with sleep and rest, as the earth is a quiet source of healing energy. Touch is essential for helping each other.

So much of my teachings have occurred in Ceremony close to the earth. We honour the earth during the harvest Protocol. We honour the earth as life source when we bleed our animals in the field, allowing the cycle to continue. Ceremonies such as sweat bath and Sweat Lodge for purification and prayer also occur close to the earth. These Ceremonies also combine water, air, and earth medicine, using medicinal plants and aromas to cleanse and purify and bring prayers to Creator. It is important to acknowledge the earth as the source of healing, providing energy for the plants and everything that surrounds us on this planet, and it naturally balances the air energy from above that we breathe.

Ceremony gives us opportunity for physical, emotional, and spiritual detoxification and purification. Up north, we use hot springs, banya, or sauna. Other places may use a Sweat Lodge. From the cleansing sulfur pools in the subarctic to Sweat Lodge in the desert southwest, heat is a known spiritual purifier. It helps rid the body of unnecessary weight and toxins, allowing us to sweat and detoxify our bodies, minds, and spirits. Great respect should be paid to the traditional Protocols for how long to soak or how to sweat. Sometimes a shrub switch was used during steam baths. This might include local wormwood (*Artemisia* species) or alder. Other purification methods include infusing the home with spruce needles boiled on the stove. I have known Traditional Healers to practise smudging with cedar, which is also used during a sweat. There is also a local sage (another species of *Artemisia*) that can be used for smudge, in addition to white sage (*Salvia aping*) that is originally from the California area. Get to know your local resources if you have interest in these ways. Ceremony, like those described above, is useful for stopping old habits, processing emotions, interrupting neural pathways and laying down new ones, bringing balance to energy circuits, and clearing the way for a new possibility.

As a child, I looked forward to when I would be heavy enough to be able to walk on backs with enough force to help others. So many patients have complained of agonizing pain that has been debilitating for months and sometimes decades. Simple, ceremonial, hands-on treatments, alleviating congested and painful tissue, benefit patients, sometimes transforming lives in as little as one visit.

Harvesting and Preparing Foods for Health and Well-Being

Harvesting and preparing traditional foods in our communities gives form to our bodies, and feeds our mind and spirit as seasons pass. We have a spiritual connection to earth as Athabascan people, and we recognize the kingdoms of the plants, animals, insects, and minerals. In the modern setting, it is unlikely to be able to live a completely traditional diet. However, using modern techniques, we can continue to expand our use of plants and plant medicines, adding to our traditional diet.

Food is central to our survival in the remote north, and with limited access to greens in the winter, we are grateful for the animals who offer themselves. When we harvest our first animal, we show respect by honouring the animal in prayer or Ceremony at the time of harvest. The first harvest is prepared and shared with family, particularly Elders, signifying the importance of our interconnectedness and gratitude for the earth that provides.

Traditional diets had all the essential components for a balanced diet, including essential fatty acids, antioxidants, calories and protein, and many health benefits such as protection from diabetes, cardiovascular disease, improved maternal nutrition, and neonatal and infant brain development (Egeland, Feyk, and Middaugh 1998). However, as animals can bioaccumulate toxins, we must be cautious with our traditional foods, especially seal oil and predator fish, which have high levels of toxins (Dewailly et al. 1993). A healthy diet is one where a variety of simple, natural ingredients our grandparents would recognize as food are enjoyed calmly in company, and thoroughly chewed and digested. However, we must choose with some awareness of our changing times. We can only do so much to modify our diet, and the time has come to minimize toxicity to our environment and consider whether our health is a priority globally.

Basic guidelines include eating a rainbow variety of foods including mostly veggies, roots, and healthy fats such as seeds, nuts, or wild meats instead of processed boxed foods engineered to last but not nourish. This allows us exposure to a maximum variety of nutrients and other constituents in food that promote health. An example of a variety of traditional foods might include cranberries and blueberries mixed with white bear fat, sautéed brown wild mushrooms, with dried fish and boiled fish eggs with fermented greens. Traditional diets included a wide variety of foods, such as naturally rendered fats, bone broth, and aged and fermented foods that are not widely used today.

Minimizing exposure to potentially toxic foods such as processed meat, widely available in grocery stores today, could benefit us. The International Agency for Research on Cancer published a press release confirming that processed meat is a human carcinogen and causes colorectal cancer (IARC 2015). Processed meats can be described as bacon, sausages, hot dogs, ham, salami, pepperoni, but not fresh meats. Traditionally, meats were dried, and sometimes salt was used, but this is quite different from the intensive processing that these products undergo. We continue to eat toxic processed meats and too much sugar, despite much evidence showing their toxic effects.

Traditional diets also included animal proteins like fish. Fish oil has become well known for health benefits. These amazing ancient creatures are central to our diet and lifestyle on the Yukon River. Like the fish, we migrate, from winter to summer camp. Now we look forward to their arrival, and they sustain us through the dark winters with their delicious, healthy nutrients. Early studies showed that Greenlandic Inuit peoples, who ate primarily from the sea, had low rates of cardiovascular disease (Dyerberg, Bang, and Hjørne 1975). Many studies have looked at the health benefits of fish oil (Howard et al. 2009; Kar and Webel 2012). In particular, pregnant ladies and young children could benefit. Those with inflammatory or mental or emotional complaints can also use fish oil as medicine. The human brain contains 60 per cent fat, thus it is vital to pay attention to fats in our diet, and especially the quality of the fats makes a difference (Chang, Ke, and Chen 2009). Be sure to consider molecularly distilled or pharmaceutical-grade fish oil that removes mercury, and stop taking one week prior to medical procedures as it thins the blood.

Fats are essential for optimum health, however not all fats are healthful. Healthy fats contain mono- and polyunsaturated fats that provide building blocks for our bodies and have their own medicinal properties. Polyunsaturated fatty acids are found in wild game. We traditionally render fats, and use the fats to deliver plant medicine by heating the oil and plant together, being careful to not burn the oil. These medicines have been used for generations. Plants also contain oils mostly in their seeds. Examples of healthy oils include avocado, olive oil, and nuts, which have monounsaturated fatty acids. In the modern era, traditional diets have largely replaced our consumption of healthy fats with sugars. Unhealthy fats include trans-fats and partially hydrogenated fats. These fats occur in small amounts in meats, but are lower in traditional meats. Modern food industry changes the chemical structure of the fats to "hydrogenate" them, and thus add shelf life, flavour, and texture to processed foods. These are well known to increase cholesterol and poorly impact health, while increasing our risk for diabetes and heart disease (Liu et al. 2018; Wang and Hu 2017). These artificial fats are added to foods such as peanut butter to keep oils from separating at room temperature. Be sure to check labels when eating nut butters and packaged foods to avoid added trans fats, especially those that are hydrogenated, to minimize your risk of developing chronic disease.

For as long as we can remember, we have been drinking bone broth to stave off famine and as medicine for those needing to rest their bodies and recuperate, such as after hard work or delivery of babies. When animals graze on the land, they absorb the minerals and nutrients from this land that has sustained our ancestors for millennia. Consider utilizing bones from large-boned four-leggeds, smaller-boned birds and mammals, or fish. Generally, the fine fish bones are cooked for a shorter duration than the larger bones. I also find pressure cooking fish with the bones in is a fantastic source of calcium. When making bone broth, I roast the bones first for forty-five minutes at 375°F (190°C). I was told this causes cracks in the bony matrix and improves the leeching of minerals into the broth.

I recall stories of Elders pulverizing bones to ensure every nutrient possible was boiled and eaten. We believe bone broth is helpful for promoting overall health through nourishment, and providing minerals especially when fasting due to prolonged illness, or fasting with bone broth as a treatment for chronic illness. I would consider encouraging those at risk for, or with, the following complaints to consider consuming bone broth:

osteoporosis, digestive problems, muscle aches or cramps, chronic joint pain, nerve problems, intestinal complaints, brittle nails, and hair thinning. The following is my bone broth recipe.

Bone Broth Recipe

4 pieces of bone about 20 cm long, such as leg bone (or more if you like)—preferably from free-range, organically raised, or wild large animals such as moose or caribou

1 celery heart (or 3 ribs)

3 large carrots, roughly chopped

4 onions, chopped in half

1 bunch of greens (parsley, cilantro, nettle, seaweed, whatever you would like)

4 litres of water

Directions

1. Combine ingredients in large stockpot, and cover with water and bring to boil.
2. Then allow to simmer for 3–8 hours. Though some people simmer for up to 24 hours. Bones have been saved and reused in the past.
3. Filter or scoop out the solids, and enjoy the broth freshly cooked, or place in containers and freeze for later use.

In addition to bone broth, traditional diets included fermented foods. Our most well known fermented foods include stink fish, or stink flipper, allowing us to soften parts that would be otherwise hard to eat and preserve foods for consuming later. However, many different kinds of fermented foods are available, or can be made. These include traditional greens lightly fermented in water, as well as those from other cultures such as kefir, yogurt, sauerkraut, kombucha, miso, and kimchi. Fermented foods were common in the traditional Alaska Native diet, and are essential to help maintain healthy gut balance. A review article published in the *Journal of Applied Microbiology* (Parvez et al. 2006) found multiple health benefits from fermented food products, including improved intestinal tract health, enhanced immune function, increased synthesis of nutrients, and increased bioavailability of nutrients, meaning that available nutrients can be taken up into the body. Symptoms of lactose intolerance, such as bloating and diarrhea after eating cow dairy, diminished after consuming ferments. Additionally, the prevalence of allergy and risk of certain cancers was reduced from consuming fermented food products. Our people have Protocols for specific foods, including the manner in which to prepare them and exact ways of place and time for fermentation. Now is the time to safely learn with an expert and pass on our knowledge.

We must follow specific Protocols carefully to adopt new technologies. Recent practices of fermenting in plastic containers, as opposed to in the earth, limit access to air and oxygen. Thus, an illness called botulism can occur. We see botulism when folks experience tingling and nerve problems such as paralysis after eating foods that have been improperly fermented, promoting toxin production from the bacteria. This simply underlines the importance of following traditional Protocols that did not include plastic containers in the fermentation process. This information is summarized nicely in the State of Alaska Department of Health and Human Services (DHHS) *Botulism in Alaska Monograph*, updated in November 2017.

The following five food safety steps are recommended by the Centers for Disease Control and Prevention and DHHS for persons who prepare or eat traditional aged foods:

1. Try to use traditional methods for preparing Alaska Native foods, as these may decrease the likelihood the food will become contaminated with botulism bacteria. Plastic, glass, or sealed plastic bags do not allow air to reach the food and can promote the growth of *Clostridium botulinum* bacteria. Use salt to preserve dried fish and to also discourage growth of *C. botulinum* bacteria.

2. Age food at a cold temperature, ideally below 36° Fahrenheit (or 2° Celsius). This will also discourage the growth of *C. botulinum* bacteria.

3. Before preparing food, wash your hands, your containers, and your food.

4. Cook your food before eating it. Heat destroys *botulinum* toxin, and may be the best way to reduce the risk of getting botulism after eating aged foods.

5. When in doubt, throw it out! Don't take the risk of getting botulism if you don't know how the food was prepared. *Botulinum* toxin is so deadly, even a small taste can make you ill.

High-quality fat served as the main source of calories in the traditional diet. The modern diet has largely replaced calories from healthy fat with processed sugars. Historically, we had only seasonal exposure to sweet berries and greens with carbohydrates. There was an extended time without these delicacies during our long winters. Now we consume more sugar than ever before, and this has tremendous adverse health effects. As illustrated in Figure 13.1, sugar consumption per individual has greatly increased. Researchers have examined trends in sugar consumption over time, and the increase in chronic disease rates, including obesity, hypertension, metabolic syndrome, type 2 diabetes, and kidney disease. They explore the possibility that sugar intake, particularly a specific sugar, fructose, as contributing to prevalence of chronic illness.

This graph illustrates that as sugar from cane and beet processing become more widely available globally, we have experienced an increase in chronic maladies. This is particularly notable after the development of high-fructose corn syrup introduced in the United States in the early 1970s. Specifically, sugar and high-fructose corn syrup (highly processed sugar) have resulted in an additional 30 per cent increase in overall sweetener intake over the past forty years, mostly in the form of soft drinks (Johnson et al. 2007).

People in Western countries are consuming massive amounts of refined sugars, reaching about 150 lbs (67 kg) per year in some countries (USDA 2021; OECD 2015, Table A.12.2; Cordain et al. 2005). This amounts to over five hundred calories of sugar per day. Our bodies do not need excess sugar, and it is much less healthful than if we eat healthy mono- and polyunsaturated fats such as are found in traditional foods such as moose, caribou, bear, beaver, and fish (Clifton and Keogh 2017). It is very clear that we are consuming way more sugar than our bodies are equipped to handle (Welsh et al. 2011).

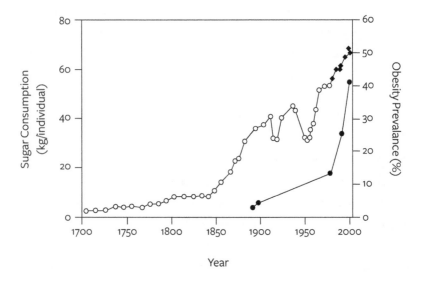

FIGURE 13.1 *Sugar intake per capita in the United Kingdom (1700–1978) and in the United States (1975–2000) is compared with obesity rates in the United States in non-Hispanic white men aged 60–69. Values for 1880 to 1910 are based on studies conducted in male Civil War veterans aged 50–59 (Johnson et al. 2007, 901).*

Historically, fructose, a sugar in fruit, was available seasonally. Remember, our berries only ripen a certain time of year. I am inspired to recall my time in the Arizona desert, where I learned from the Tohono O'odham Nation to harvest the great saguaro cactus fruit. This is no easy task, considering the fruit are at the tip-top of the cactus, and must be caught when plucked with a special tool. I gained a deeper understanding of the efforts of harvest in the squelching heat, and suddenly found myself feeling lucky for easy berry harvest on the spongy tundra. Unlike glucose that can be stored in the liver and muscles as glycogen (a larger, sugar-like molecule), the fructose sugar found in fruit is converted to fat for storage. Thus, our high-fruit diets can also contribute to calorie and weight imbalance. I encourage patients to be conscious of the amount of sweets (including fruits) they consume.

Traditional fruits, especially berries, which require community ties, tradition, and lots of work to harvest, are best. Also of note, they are particularly low in fructose. Our fruits grow close to the ground in Alaska, and the berries are strong medicine.

Plant Medicine

I was taught that Mother Earth is a source of life and can be medicine, though ultimately healing comes from our connection to our higher power. Traditionally, our people understood that certain plants close to the earth take on this powerful quality. Blueberries and cranberries are examples that are helpful for urinary complaints, healthy vessels especially in the eyes, and cough and cold complaints. And dandelion root is a surprisingly strong and helpful medicine. My teachers say that our medicines are stronger due to the harsh environment, and that the fresh and harsher air in the mountains and on the coast enhances the medicines. Alaskan blueberries have been found to have twice the level of disease-fighting antioxidants compared with commercial blueberries, corroborating our use of them as medicine (Grace et al. 2014).

I have included a brief overview and summary of plant medicine teachings, and discuss three powerful plant medicines for detoxification and health. These include stinging nettle, dandelion, and blueberry. It is important to know our own limitations and familiarize yourself with resources to ask for help. Be aware of your own limits with plant medicines, whether you are new to them, or even if they are old friends. Below, I provide a general list of cautions for plant medicine. I always encourage patients and herbalists to work in conjunction with health care providers when caring for patients.

Cautions with Plant Medicine

1. Apply caution when treating yourself and others with plants as medicine.
2. Know your limits, and refer to experts when necessary.
3. Please be considerate that not all medicines or plants may be safe, and many have toxic constituents. I find it helpful to know the plants that are poisonous where I am harvesting, as some plants can toxify their neighbours.

4. Pregnant women, breastfeeding women, and children need particular caution, as do the elderly and those on Western medications.
5. Please consult local experts. There is no replacement for hands-on learning from Elders and experts.
6. Work with medical providers and pharmacists who have access to herb-drug interactions and can advise and monitor for interactions. Be aware that we just don't have data for all traditional herbs and pharmaceuticals.
7. Be aware of allergies.
8. Follow the Protocol for harvesting plants.

Be sure to minimize toxin exposure when harvesting. Think about and know about the natural processes: wind patterns, tides, watersheds, and river routes that may contribute to distributing toxins. Avoid gathering in polluted areas, and plants that show stress or damage.

Plant Harvest Protocol

There is a Protocol for plant harvesting that I feel blessed to share. You may have your own Protocols that are different and that contribute to the balance and complex nature of our relationship with the earth. Hunting, gathering, and trade networks continue to exist. This local knowledge allows us to gather with the seasons, reaping the benefits at peak ripeness and nutritional value. We must continue to value and pass those harvesting Protocols on to our next generation.

1. Harvest with gratitude and respect.
2. Ask the plants for permission by assessing the health of the plant population and looking if the area is safe and healthy for harvest.
3. Offer Ceremony to honour the plants and their sacrifice performed. This is not always done when gathering foods, however, when using plants for medicine, this is important. We pray for the people or illnesses we plan to treat. If the root of the plant needs to be taken, special attention is paid, sometimes spending the night outside with the plant, as the life of the plant will be taken.

4. A gift such as tobacco, a bead, a strand of hair, or a song is offered out of gratitude, respect, and interconnection.

5. Do not harvest after dark, so as to not disturb or offend these beings.

6. Ensure a clean and quick cut with a sharp knife or scissors across the appropriate plant part, and be careful to not pick more than you need or can process. Pick sparingly, taking only what you need (some say 10–20 per cent of the plant community).

Some Plant Medicines

Stinging Nettle, Urtica dioica

Introduction

Used traditionally from Ireland to Alaska. Local Dena'ina use this mineral-dense plant for food, adding them to stews and fish dishes. Traditional name: "that which stings." They have ragged leaf edges.

Food Uses: The shoots and young leaves are edible, however do not eat when mature. Gather with gloves. Cook like spinach. Cook, juice, freeze, or dry to denature the sting (Krohn 2007).

Other Uses: Remarkably, the fibre from nettles can be spun as twine to make fibre, blankets, and nets.

Medicinal Uses: Used for rheumatism; people applied leaves around the inflamed joint.

Medicinal Properties: Monitor blood clotting (international normalized ratio if anticoagulation), has anti-inflammatory, diuretic, and healthy prostate (benign prostatic hyperplasia) properties.

Harvest: Wear gloves to pick shoots and leaves in the spring. Caution: When harvesting nettle to eat fresh, collect prior to flowering. Older leaves contain cystoliths, thought to possibly irritate the kidney. The stinging compound is denatured by drying and heating.

Preparation for Tea: 1 tbsp/cup boiled water, steep fifteen minutes, drink up to several times a day.

Contraindications:
- cardiac failure;
- renal failure.

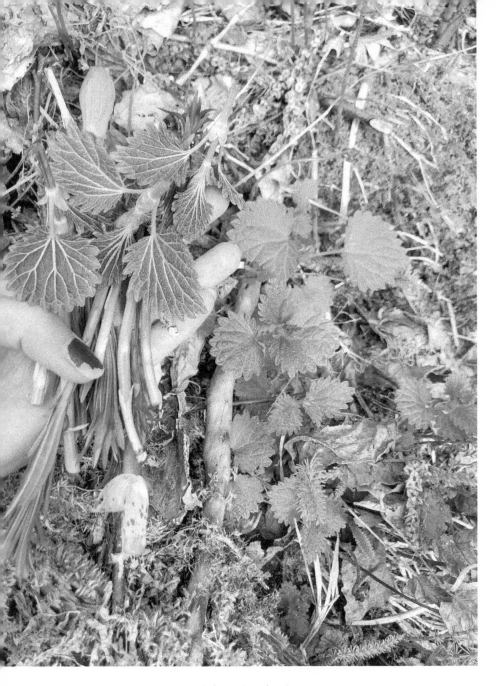

FIGURE 13.2 *Stinging nettle* (Urtica dioica) *in the spring.*
[*Photo by Allison Kelliher, used with permission.*]

Medication Side Effects/Medicine Interactions:

- dyspepsia/nausea, topical irritation;
- may increase effect of diclofenac (NSAID[1]) (Johnson 2002).

Stinging Nettle Contents:

- antioxidants;
- vitamins and minerals (vitamins A, C, D; iron, calcium, potassium, magnesium, manganese);
- nutrients (protein, chlorophyll) (Gray 2012, 420).

Dandelion, Taraxacum officinale

Introduction

Dandelion is a powerful plant with multiple uses and is powerful medicine. It so often is thought of as a nuisance. I have learned there are local and introduced dandelion, and all are medicinal. My teachers encourage me to listen to the plants, and that the dandelion is here to help us detox our modern lifestyle. It has bitter properties that prepare our digestive enzymes to digest food, and inulin, which is a prebiotic. Additionally, it is considered safe for human consumption as a food by the United States Food and Drug Administration (USDA 2019). It has history of use as a folk and traditional remedy in Costa Rica, Mexico, Canada, and the United States. It is in the sunflower family but is also related to ragweed, so beware if you have an allergy to that.

Food Uses: It can be used as salad greens, and in soups, wine, and teas.
It is so generous in that you can harvest something from it from spring to fall. When roasted, the root is used as a coffee substitute.

Medicinal Uses: The roasted root can be used in treatment of diabetes.
The root is a diuretic, so be mindful of dosing earlier in the day.

Harvest: Leaves are preferable before blooming; they become bitter; you can harvest flowers and roots (in spring or fall). Fall roots are sweeter with more inulin. Use caution if you have a ragweed allergy.

Contraindications:

- biliary obstruction/stone;
- intestinal obstruction.

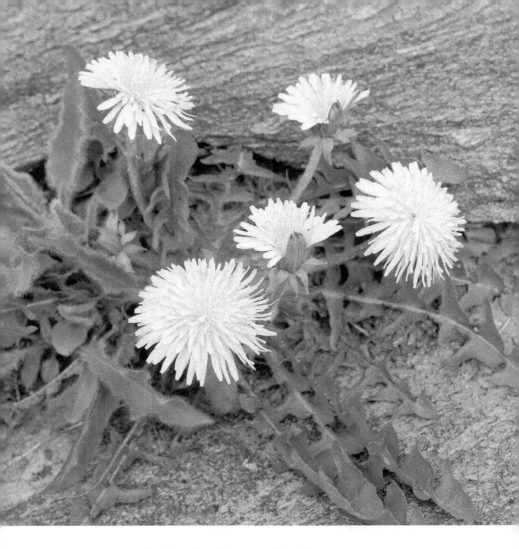

FIGURE 13.3 *Dandelion flower* (Taraxacum officinale).
[Photo by Randi Hausken. Used under Creative Commons licence 2.0.
https://flickr.com/photos/randihausken/3483575184/in/photostream/.]

Medication Side Effects/Medicine Interactions:
· allergic reaction, biliary inflammation, biliary obstruction, dermatitis,
  may increase effects of some diuretics;
· quinolone antibiotics: may decrease effectiveness;
· lithium—diuretic-like—may decrease levels;

- cytochrome P450 1A2 (CYP1A2) substrates: amitriptyline, haloperidol, ondansetron, propranolol, theophylline, verapamil, and others;
- glucuronidated drugs: acetaminophen, atorvastatin, diazepam, digoxin, entacapone, estrogen, irinotecan, lamotrigin, lorazepam, lovastatin (Mevacor), meprobamate, morphine, oxazepam, and others (Blumenthal, Goldberg, and Brinckmann 2000, 78–83).

Dandelion Contents:

- vitamins and minerals (B vitamins, vitamins A, C, D; calcium, copper, iron, magnesium, manganese, potassium, selenium, silicon, and zinc) (Gray 2012, 420).

Blueberry, Vaccinium *spp*

Introduction

Blueberries are often referred to as a superfood due to their high nutritional content and medicinal value. We gather the berries and the plant to eat and make a tea as a tonic to prevent disease. Blueberries and their cousin, cranberry, are *Vaccinium* species. They are known to be rich in antioxidants, including anthocyanins, which are known to protect against neurodegeneration that leads to diseases such as dementia (Jong 2013). They are eaten when in season and frozen in quantity. Traditional Healers use the medicine for people who are at risk for diabetes, have diabetes, or complain of sore varicose veins. There appears to be benefit from consuming approximately 1/3 cup a day of blueberries.

Food Uses: We love our blueberries, and prepare them in many ways including fresh, dried, with cream, in sauces, jellies, jams, and deserts. They can also be mixed with meat and fat into pemmican. And they have been used for pickling fish and on bearded seal meat (Krohn 2007).

Other Uses: Blueberry has been used as a dye for baskets, skins, and quills (Krohn 2007).

Medicinal Uses: Blueberries and other plants are filled with vitamins, nutrients, and phytomedicines that promote wellness. They contain astringent tannins that have anti-inflammatory properties. There is evidence for potential benefit for age-related diseases such as

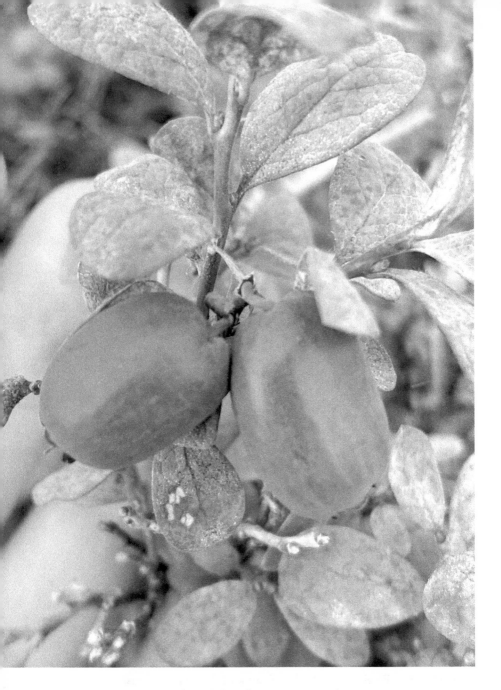

FIGURE 13.4 *Bog or alpine blueberry* (Vaccinium uiginosum*).*

[*Photo by Allison Kelliher, used with permission.*]

dementia, vessel health effecting vision and varicosities, and diabetes mellitus type 2. Other medical indications include cystitis, urethritis, and hypoglycemia (Schofield 1989, 81). Schofield (1989) recommends you start slow on the tea, as there are some reports of toxicity with consuming a lot of tea. According to the American Botanical Council (Blumenthal, Goldberg, and Brinckmann 2000), blueberry leaf tea is a safe blood sugar regulator. They recommend one cup twice a day for at least three months. It is high in anthocyanin, protecting cells from oxidative damage. Also of note, blueberry's relative bilberry contains bioflavonoids that strengthen capillaries and decrease capillary permeability, explaining some if its benefits for vessels and varicosities. Both the fruit and the leaf of bilberry and blueberry are historically used.

How to Make Medicine:

- 1/3–1 cup fresh fruit per day;
- for berry tea, simmer 2 tbsp dried berries in 2 cups water;
- for leaf tea, place 1 oz of dried leaves (3 oz fresh) in 2 cups of hot water, cover for 10 minutes (drink 1 cup up to twice a day as needed);
- extracts: dose range 360–600 mg/day standardized to 25 per cent anthocyanosides;
- tinctures are made from the leaves (apple cider-based, or alcohol-based extracts).

Harvest: The leaves are harvested in spring and early summer, while the fruits are gathered in late summer and fall.

Contraindications:

- antithrombotic agents

Medication Side Effects/Medicine Interactions:

- no significant adverse reactions noted, though may increase effects of antithrombotic agents (Johnson 2002).

Blueberry Contents:

- vitamins and minerals (B vitamins, vitamins A, C, E, K; calcium, iron, magnesium, manganese, potassium, phosphorous, sodium, and zinc) (Gray 2012, 420).

Traditional Lifestyles and Health

People with traditional lifestyles know that nature is essential for health. Traditions require physical activity for harvesting and preparation. Walking, reaching, bending, pulling, and carrying all require strength and endurance. Being active on the earth helps us to maintain balance to continue to harvest foods and medicines that our bodies and families need. Time spent in nature with natural elements has become more limited since transitioning to post-colonial times. There are health benefits to being in nature, and we are more likely to care for nature if we are in close relationship with this source of life.

Being outdoors is essential for a healthy and whole self. Consider spending as much time as you can in green or natural places, and incorporate natural elements into your homes and workplaces when possible. These places soothe our souls and expose our mind, body, and spirit to a source of rejuvenation. Studies now support that nature is medicine.

Often physical work comes seasonally. Spring is a time of great activity, releasing the stagnancy of winter, and the flurry of summer seems to pass in a blur as we prepare for autumn's harvest and rest again in the winter. There are challenges to maintaining an active lifestyle year-round as the weather, facilities, and time all limit access to recreational space. Simple body move-ment such as walking, even in place, is a great way to move year-round. Simply walking and standing daily can have tremendous benefit for patients I see who have complaints of mood (anxiety and depression), and pain due to stiffness and arthritis. Bodies need movement and full breath to lubricate joints and tissues for optimum health. Dr. Levine is a researcher at the Mayo Clinic and the National Institutes of Health. He reports that sitting too much leads to more than thirty chronic diseases contributing to high health care costs. He encourages us to reimagine how we can incorporate movement into our schools, work environments, and community (Levine 2015). Traditionally, our lifestyles were active, as we lived off the land following the herds of caribou. Modern lifestyles create a sedentary setting, where all the sitting we do is just as bad for us as smoking cigarettes.

If we care for our bodies, our bodies will take care of us, and we in turn will foster a deeper relationship with Earth and be better equipped to take care of her, the source of life. Translating this into my life and practice, I find it helpful to ask people what they enjoy to address barriers to activity. Some folks love walking on the trails, and others would rather walk on an even surface at the mall. It is very important that we learn to listen to our body and not overdo activity and cause unnecessary wear and tear. I encourage a variety of activities, including walking, stretching, tai chi, yoga, biking, hiking, hunting, ice fishing, skiing, ice-skating, swimming, housecleaning, and gardening—anything that gets us moving.

The World Health Organization (WHO) has created a summary of activity to prevent developing chronic disease in adults up to sixty-four years of age (WHO 2020):

- Minimum of 150 minutes of moderate-intensity aerobic physical activity per week.
- Aerobic activity performed in bouts of at least ten minutes duration (high heart rate, high-intensity exercise).
- Muscle-strengthening activities for major muscle groups two or more days a week.

Natural elements such as a view outside and exposure to light improve health outcomes in hospitals. Bright daytime light improves outcomes in hospitals by reducing length of stay. Both patients and staff satisfaction improve with access to sunlight (Swan, Richardson, and Hutton 2003). According to a randomized controlled trial conducted at the Department of Neuropsychiatric Sciences at the University of Milan, bipolar patients assigned to rooms with more sunlight had a mean 3.67-day shorter hospital stay than patients with the same who did not have sunlight (Benedetti et al. 2001). It is particularly effective when applied in the morning and for those with a mental health diagnosis. It was found to be helpful in reducing depression among hospitalized patients with bipolar disorder or seasonal affective disorders (Benedetti et al. 2001; Beauchemin and Hays 1996; Wallace-Guy et al. 2002). A randomized control test conducted by Columbia University found that bright light is an effective antidepressant in patients with seasonal affective disorder (Terman, Terman, and Ross 1998). Other studies have demonstrated the negative effects of windowless hospital rooms on outcomes and satisfaction, demonstrating high rates of anxiety, depression, and delirium without exposure to natural light (Keep 1977). In addition to improving these outcomes, sun exposure on the skin activates the essential hormone vitamin D, which is necessary for a healthy skeletal and immune system.

Time in Nature is essential for us to connect to the source of life and learn to care for her as she cares for us. Nature exposure benefits us, and also fosters a need for us to care for the earth. The following studies take a closer look at our most precious resource, children, and how nature affects their behaviour and development.

Proven Benefits of Regular Play in Nature

Children who play in more natural environments develop advanced coordination, balance, and social environments that can buffer stress. Knowing about this can help us build resiliency by encouraging us to find and participate in our communities and nurture companionship and friendships. For as long as I can remember, my family harvests together. Harvesting large game and substantial quantities of berries are examples of a traditional lifestyle that requires we have many hands and minds. This includes teachers and also those who are learning, so we can help each other along the way. The benefits of companionship have been evidenced in animal studies looking at stress hormones produced by lab mice. When the mice were stressed, they produced a predictable hormone response. However, when they had a companion, their stress response was negligible (Levine 1997). It turns out that spending time with each other is a great healing asset.

Studies have confirmed that support during times of illness enhances health. Family visits to hospitalized patients provide a form of social support that can help to alleviate the effects of stress that can arise with an illness or associated hospitalization. Several studies addressed whether family involvement or interactions affected patient outcomes during hospital stays. One study concluded that family presence during invasive procedures in the pediatric intensive care unit decreased procedure-related anxiety (Powers and Rubenstein 1999). Several studies also found that there are barriers to involving families and social support networks during a patient's hospital stay, such as restricted visiting hours or a lack of beds or rooms where parents can stay with hospitalized children (Benians 1988; Walker 1998). According to the literature, single rooms allow for increased privacy and confidentiality, as well as decreased stress for family, staff, and patients. And there is some evidence showing that our strong social support system may be contributing to increased feelings of love, contentment, and optimism, as well as reducing our stress hormone, cortisol (Luks 1988). This is important to consider in our healing settings of today and in the future so we are able to utilize the health benefits of community and support each other's health.

We are connected to the previous generations. Being born into a place that we know and feel kinship with, we are often gifted names reflecting those who held respect and knowledge. We receive graciously from the land and water that has nourished our peoples for as many generations as we can recall. This is balanced reciprocally by giving back to the land with stewardship, awareness, and conscious harvest and use of the interconnected miraculous bounty.

Today's fast-pace, instant-gratification, superficial, commodity-based popular culture threatens the very lifeblood of existence on the planet— poisoning the sacred with artificial additives and polluting our air and breath. Our ancestors have spoken of this for generations, and our voice is still heard and still needs to be heard. Unpredictable storms, water levels rising, unpredictable harvests, and violence threaten people every day. It is so important to remember the ways to bring harmony and balance back into our daily lives.

Change seems the only constant. Changing cycles on the earth—I was born into a time when the Bering Sea froze over completely, such that dogsled races were run across it. Now the ice is not dependable, and we cannot rely on leaving. A late and new species of hummingbird stayed well into November in Anchorage, Alaska! It proved to be the Costa's hummingbird, normally found in southwestern deserts. This creates a unique challenge for those of us in northern climates. We must adapt.

As chronic disease prevalence across the world increases, we are obligated to consider all potentially successful treatments. Chronic diseases are expensive and complex to manage. Traditional Alaska Native healing and other global healing traditions can serve as a resource to help solve these problems. The World Health Organization lists chronic diseases as a concern for global health. These noncommunicable diseases cause forty-one million deaths annually. In order to decrease this staggering sum, the WHO encourages a comprehensive approach. One where we work together in community to include health, finance, foreign affairs, education, agriculture, planning, and others to reduce the risks and promote prevention (WHO 2021). Further, in a separate report (Alderete 1999), the WHO informed us that Traditional Healing systems co-exist with Western medicine in all regions of the world, providing primary sources of care for up to 80 per cent of the population in developing countries. This creates a unique opportunity for Indigenous communities to remember and continue to practise our healing ways.

In America, we have an increasing reliance on pharmaceuticals (Kantor et al. 2015). And, despite this, our disease burdens continue to skyrocket. According to the Centers for Disease Control and Prevention (2021), chronic diseases are responsible for seven of ten deaths each year, and treating people with chronic diseases accounts for 86 per cent of our nation's health care costs. So, when you think about it, Traditional Healers are perfectly poised for a revolution in health care and health care delivery. It could be of great benefit for us to remember the very basics of being well that prior generations employed. The importance of changing the unhealthy behaviours that underlie pathology are paramount. If we employed appropriate lifestyle changes, 93 per cent of diabetes mellitus type 2, 81 per cent of heart attacks, 50 per cent of strokes, and 36 per cent of cancers would be prevented. These changes include healthy nutrition, a balance of exercise and rest, stress management, social integration, appropriate exposure to a clean environment, no smoking, moderate alcohol consumption, and no or limited exposure to toxic chemicals (Ford et al. 2009).

Despite these challenges, it is important to see the berry bucket as being half-full, rather than half-empty. Optimism is clearly linked to happier and more satisfying romantic relationships due to greater cooperative problem solving (Assad et al. 2007). Traditional Healing ways offer many options for treating complex lifestyle diseases. We can offer a range of options not limited to traditional counselling, dietary guidance with cultural relevance, energy medicine (calming and relieves pain), and touch therapies (specific techniques for releasing or relaxing blockages, including in microsystems such as the feet). Recent research encouraged pediatricians to evaluate the level of clinical risk that the chosen therapy might pose. Further, it encourages shared decision making, while continuing to monitor conventionally and being prepared to intervene when medically required. The pediatricians' primary concerns are use of dangerous treatments and over reliance on alternative treatments, while excluding potentially beneficial therapies (see Cohen 2006).

Closing Reflection

Live simply and employ the ancient knowledge of our ancestors. Science now confirms and supports our traditional lifeway. Just as the salmon returns to the source at the end of life, we are returning to a time when we must remember and honour the original instructions for how to be human. This will help to restore our basic sources of health. Air, water, and earth allow us to exist and combine to inspire an opportunity each moment for us to recreate a state of balance. We have much work to do helping each other to remember and practise healthy lifeways. I encourage you to listen with your heart and follow what you hear.

NOTE

1.	NSAIDs are nonsteroidal, anti-inflammatory drugs, including Aspirin and Ibuprofen, as well as other compounds. Diclofenac is an NSAID.

REFERENCES

Alaska Department of Health and Human Services (DHHS). 2017. *Botulism in Alaska Monograph*. November 2017. http://dhss.alaska.gov/dph/Epi/id/Pages/botulism/resources.aspx.

Alderete E.W. 1991. *The Health of Indigenous Peoples*. Geneva: World Health Organization.

Assad, K., M. Assad, B. Donnellan, and R.D. Conge. 2007. "Optimism: An Enduring Resource for Romantic Relationships." *Journal of Personality and Social Psychology* 93, no 2: 285–97.

Barati, F., A. Nasiri, N. Akbari, and G. Sharifzadeh. 2016. "The Effect of Aromatherapy on Anxiety in Patients." *Nephrourology Monthly* 8, no. 5: e38347.

Beauchemin, K.M., and P. Hays. 1996. "Sunny Hospital Rooms Expedite Recovery from Severe and Refractory Depressions." *Journal of Affective Disorders* 40, no. 1–2: 49–51.

Benedetti, F., C. Colombo, B. Barbini, E. Campori, and E. Smeraldi. 2001. "Morning Sunlight Reduces Length of Hospitalization in Bipolar Depression." *Journal of Affective Disorders* 62, no. 3: 221–23.

Benians, R.C. 1988. "The Influence of Parental Visiting on Survival and Recovery of Extensively Burned Children." *Burns* 14, no. 1: 31–34.

Blumenthal, M., A. Goldberg, and J. Brinckmann, eds. 2000. *Herbal Medicine Expanded Commission E Monographs*. Austin, Texas: American Botanical Council.

Brown, R.P., and P.L. Gerbarg. 2005. "Sudarshan Kriya Yogic Breathing in the Treatment of Stress, Anxiety, and Depression." *The Journal of Alternative and Complementary Medicine* 11, no. 4: 711–17.

Brownfield, A. 1998. "Aromatherapy in Arthritis: A Study." *Nursing Standard* 13, no. 5: 34–35.

Buckle, J. 1999. "Use of Aromatherapy as a Complementary Treatment for Chronic Pain." *Alternative Therapies in Health and Medicine* 5, no. 5: 42–51.

Centers for Disease Control and Prevention (CDC). 2021. *Mortality in the United States, 2020*. NCHS Data Brief No. 427, December 2021. https://www.cdc.gov/nchs/products/databriefs/db427.htm.

Chang, C.Y., D.S. Ke, and J.Y. Chen. 2009. "Essential Fatty Acids and Human Brain." *Acta Neurol Taiwan* 18, no. 4: 231–41.

Clifton, P.M., and J.B. Keogh. 2017. "A Systematic Review of the Effect of Dietary Saturated and Polyunsaturated Fat on Heart Disease." *Nutrition, Metabolism and Cardiovascular Diseases* 27, no. 12: 1060–80.

Cohen, M. 2006. "Legal and Ethical Issues Relating to Use of Complementary Therapies in Pediatric Hematology/Oncology." *Journal of Pediatric Hematology/Oncology* 28, no. 3: 190–93.

Cordain, L., S. Boyd Eaton, A. Sebastian, N. Mann, S. Lindeberg, B.A. Watkins, J.H. O'Keefe, et al. 2005. "Origins and Evolution of the Western Diet: Health Implications for the 21st Century." *The American Journal of Clinical Nutrition* 81, no. 2: 341–54. https://doi.org/10.1093/ajcn.81.2.341.

Dewailly, E., P. Ayotte, S. Bruneau, C. Laliberté, D.C. Muir, and R.J. Norstrom. 1993. "Inuit Exposure to Organichlorines through the Aquatic Food Chain in Arctic Quebec." *Environmental Health Perspectives* 101, no. 7: 618–20.

Dyerberg J., H.O. Bang, and N. Hjørne. 1975. "Fatty Acid Composition of the Plasma Lipids in Greenland Eskimos." *The American Journal of Clinical Nutrition* 28, no. 9: 958–66.

Egeland, G., L.A. Feyk, and J.P. Middaugh. 1998. *The Use of Traditional Foods in a Healthy Diet in Alaska*. Section of Epidemiology, Alaska Division of Public Health. January 15, 1998.

Ford, E.S., M.M. Bergmann, J. Kröger, A. Schienkiewitz, C. Weikert, and H. Boeing. 2009. "Healthy Living Is the Best Revenge: Findings from the European Prospective Investigation into Cancer and Nutrition-Potsdam Study." *Archives of Internal Medicine* 169, no. 15: 1355–62.

Fortuine, R. 1989. *Chills and Fever: Health and Disease in the Early History of Alaska*. Fairbanks: University of Alaska Press.

Grace, M.H., D. Esposito, K.L. Dunlap, and M.A. Lila. 2014. "Comparative Analysis of Phenolic Content and Profile, Antioxidant Capacity and Anti-inflammatory Bioactivity in Wild Alaskan and Commercial *Vaccinium* Berries." *Journal of Agricultural Food Chemistry* 62, no. 18: 4007–17.

Gray, B. 2012. *The Boreal Herbal*. Whitehorse, YT: Aroma Borealis.

Howard, B.V., A. Comuzzie, R.B. Devereux, S.O.E. Ebbesson, R.R. Fabsitz, W.J. Howard, S. Laston, et al. 2009. "Cardiovascular Disease Prevalence and Its Relation to Risk Factors in Alaska Eskimos." *Nutritional, Metabolic and Cardiovascular Disease* 20, no. 5: 350–58.

International Agency for Research on Cancer (IARC). Press Release. World Health Organization. http://www.iarc.fr/.

Itai, T., H. Amayasu, M. Kuribayashi, N. Kawamura, M. Okada, A. Momose, T. Tateyama, et al. 2000. "Psychological Effects of Aromatherapy on Chronic Hemodialysis Patients." *Psychiatry and Clinical Neurosciences* 54: 393–97.

Johnson, L. 2002. *Pocket Guide to Herbal Remedies*. Malden, MA: Blackwell Science.

Johnson, R.J., M.S. Segal, Y. Sautin, T. Nakagawa, D.I. Feig, D.H. Kang, M.S. Gersch, et al. 2007. "Potential Role of Sugar (Fructose) in the Epidemic of Hypertension, Obesity and the Metabolic Syndrome, Diabetes, Kidney Disease, and Cardiovascular Disease." *The American Journal of Clinical Nutrition* 86, no. 4: 899–906.

Jong, H. 2013. "Blueberry (*Vaccinium vigratum*) Leaf Extracts Protect against Aβ-induced Cytotoxicity and Cognitive Impairment." *Journal of Medicinal Food* 16, no. 11: 968–76.

Kantor, E.D., C.D. Rehm, J.S. Haas, A.T. Chan, and E.L. Giovannucci. 2015. "Trends in Presciption Drug Use among Adults in the United States from 1999–2012." *Journal of the American Medical Association* 314, no. 17: 1818–31.

Kar, S., and R. Webel. 2012. "Fish Oil Supplementation & Coronary Artery Disease: Does It Help?" *Missouri Medicine* 109, no. 2: 142–45.

Keep P.J. 1977. "Stimulus Deprivation in Windowless Rooms." *Anaesthesia* 32, no. 7: 598–602.

Klein, R. 1995. "Anatomy, Behavior, and Modern Human Origins." *Journal of World Prehistory* 9, no. 2: 167–98.

Krohn, E. 2007. *Wild Rose and Western Red Cedar: The Gifts of the Northwest Plains.* Bellingham, WA: Northwest Indian College.

Levine, J.A. 2015. "Sick of Sitting." *Diabetologia* 58, no. 8: 1751–58.

Levine, S. 1997. "Psychobiological Consequences of Social Relationships." *Annals of the New York Academy of Sciences* 807: 210–18.

Liu B., Y. Sun, L.G. Snetselaar, Q. Sun, Q. Yang, Z. Zhang, L. Liu, et al. 2018. "Association between Plasma Trans-Fatty Acid Concentrations and Diabetes in a Nationally Representative Sample of U.S. Adults." *Journal of Diabetes* 10, no. 8: 653–64.

Luks, A. 1988. "Helper's High: Volunteering Makes People Feel Good, Physically and Emotionally." *Psychology Today* 22, no. 10: 34–42.

Organisation for Economic Co-operation and Development (OECD). 2015. "Table A.12.2– Sugar Projections: Consumption, per Capita." In *OECD–FAO Agricultural Outlook 2015.* Paris: OECD Publishing. https://doi.org/10.1787/agr_outlook-2015-table135-en.

Parvez, S., K.A. Malik, S. Ah Kang, and H.Y. Kim. 2006. "Probiotics and Their Fermented Food Products Are Beneficial for Health." *Journal of Applied Microbiology* 100, no. 6: 1171–85.

Post-White, J., M.E. Kinney, K. Savik, J.B. Gau, C. Wilcox, and I. Lerner. 2003. "Therapeutic Massage and Healing Touch Improve Symptoms in Cancer." *Integrative Cancer Therapy* 2: 332–44.

Powers, K.S., and J.S. Rubenstein. 1999. "Family Presence during Invasive Procedures in the Pediatric Intensive Care Unit: A Prospective Study." *Archives of Pediatrics and Adolescent Medicine* 153, no. 9: 955–58.

Schofield, J.J. 1989. *Discovering Wild Plants: Alaska, Western Canada, the Northwest.* Portland, OR: Alaska Northwest Books.

Swan J.E., L.D. Richardson, and J.D. Hutton. 2003. "Do Appealing Hospital Rooms Increase Patient Evaluations of Physicians, Nurses, and Hospital Services?" *Health Care Management Review* 28, no. 3: 254–64.

Terman M., J.S. Terman, and D.C. Ross. 1998. "A Controlled Trial of Timed Bright Light and Negative Air Ionization for Treatment of Winter Depression." *Archives of General Psychiatry* 55, no. 10: 875–82.

US Department of Agriculture (USDA). 2021. *Food Availability (Per Capita) Data System: "Sweets."* Economic Research Service. https://www.ers.usda.gov/data-products/food-availability-per-capita-data-system/.

US Department of Agriculture (USDA). 2019. FoodData Central. Dandelion Greens, Raw. https://fdc.nal.usda.gov/fdc-app.html#/food-details/169226/nutrients.

Walker, S.B. 1998. "Neonatal Nurses' Views on the Barriers to Parenting in the Intensive Care Nursery? A National Study." *Australian Critical Care* 11, no. 3: 86–91.

Wallace-Guy, G.M., D.F. Kripke, G. Jean-Louis, R.D. Langer, J.A. Elliott, and A. Tuunainen. 2002. "Evening Light Exposure: Implications for Sleep and Depression." *Journal of the American Geriatrics Society* 50, no. 4: 738–39.

Wang, D.D., and F.B. Hu. 2017. "Dietary Fat and Risk of Cardiovascular Disease: Recent Controversies and Advances." *Annual Review of Nutrition* 37 (August 21): 423–46.

Welsh J.A., A.J. Sharma, L. Grellinger, and M.B. Vos. 2011. "Consumption of Added Sugars Is Decreasing in the U.S." *American Journal of Clinical Nutrition* 94, no. 3: 726–34.

World Health Organization (WHO). 2021. *Noncommunicable Diseases Factsheet.* April 2021. http://www.who.int/entity/mediacentre/factsheets/fs355/en/index.html.

World Health Organization (WHO). 2020. *Physical Activity Factsheet.* November 26, 2020. https://www.who.int/news-room/fact-sheets/detail/physical-activity.

14   *Paths Forward*

Concluding Words

LESLIE MAIN JOHNSON

In this book we have shared many voices and many pathways. The common goals are restoring health and well-being, and setting Indigenous communities of western Canada and Alaska on a just foundation to enable communities and individuals to flourish. Our contributors seek healthy communities based in justice, honouring traditional and sacred understandings, and fully and vibrantly participating in the life of contemporary Canada and the United States. As we have reviewed, there have been and remain tremendous challenges to achieving these goals. A number of different avenues of holistic health and well-being have been explored by our contributors. Economic well-being that does not challenge spiritual and traditional values, that does not require compromising land and local food security, remains difficult to achieve, and that must be achieved to create a firm foundation for healthy and thriving communities. And many of the health inequities and barriers to well-being are rooted in economic inequities, that is, grow out of poverty. The health of the environment can be in tension with economic development, but connections to the land are of deep importance in enabling Indigenous well-being, from spiritual connection to food traditions and access to healthy diets, as our contributors and other authors have emphasized.

We have considered Indigenous communities that are embedded in urban areas and are often fragmented, with their challenges of poverty, substance abuse, and disconnection. We also consider subpopulations that are enmeshed in the criminal justice system and seeking to achieve health in circumstances of incarceration (cf. Moise 2017). We have looked at communities that are in recovery from the multigenerational trauma imposed through residential schooling that have also suffered from barriers to family support and continuity imposed by confinement in Indian hospitals (cf. Geddes 2017). Spin-off problems like use of drugs and alcohol beget their own problems, such as FASD, as well as leading directly or indirectly to incarceration (cf. Moise 2017).

Some pathways forward show promise, though these are often bedevilled by insecure funding and inconsistent administrative and bureaucratic contexts. Maje and Maje Raider (Chapter 5) describe productive efforts in the Yukon at multifaceted healing and wellness promotion based in language and culture on the land, focused especially on women but also responsive to the needs of men. They have worked with a number of healing practitioners, both Indigenous and Western, from the psychotherapy community. Initially well funded by the Aboriginal Healing Foundation, the funding picture they describe now is much more challenging. Russell and Eagletail (Chapter 3) detail collaborations with Alberta Health in the context of clinic (Elbow River Healing Centre) and hospital, combining Ceremony and traditional medicines with other services. Russell also worked with incarcerated men at the Calgary Remand Centre, emphasizing self-knowledge and balance through traditional Blood spirituality. Auger (Chapter 4) queries how physicians can fit within a traditional understanding of healing in a hospital context, also based on experiences in Alberta.

Morgan (Chapter 6) lays out a comprehensive Gitxsan health plan based in traditional Gitxsan concepts of health and healing, which also emphasizes connection to land, traditional foods and medicines, and traditional skills and language. Her ambitious, community-based plan focused on on-the-land camps as one way forward, combining removal from community situations and being on the territories with positive skills building and counselling provided by practitioners of Self-Regulation Therapy (SRT)[1] (see also Morgan 2016). Camps were provided for women, men, and youth, enabling focus on the specific issues of each age group. The First Nations Health Authority funded this innovative health plan initiative.

A trio of chapters from Alaska shows a range of holistic perspectives, detailing the successful programs of the Alaska Tribal Health Consortium's Prevention programs (Chapter 7), an innovative Women's Rite of Passage camp (Chapter 8), and the experiences of an Indigenous (Koyukon) physician who is also qualified in several forms of alternative therapy, as well as bringing her Indigenous healing heritage into her practice (Chapter 13). Connections are evident between the Women's Rites of Passage described by DeWitt and the family healing camps on land presented by Morgan. The Alaska chapters show initiatives that have developed in the distinctive context of Alaska as part of the United States, and moving forward from the Alaska Native Claims Settlement Act.

Badry and Goose (Chapter 9) approached women's health and FASD in the Far North in Ulukhaktok, Nunavut, employing a Photovoice technique. The beautiful images shared by the women participants give a personal and intimate view of moving forward with life despite challenges. The collaboration between Badry, a "southern" social work professor from Calgary, and Goose, an Inuvialuit Elder and resident of the community, was productive and effective. Themes found in analysis of the images resonate through other contributions as well: the significance of community, family, traditions, language and crafts, and time on the land itself were all seen as important foundations for health and well-being.

Somewhat of an outlier, but spotlighting an important arena to consider in collaborative efforts to improve Indigenous community health, is the contribution by Marc Fonda (Chapter 10), who tackles the issue of Traditional Knowledge and intellectual property. The theme of concern over loss of control over traditional remedies was briefly alluded to in Russel and Eagletail's chapter, and remains a concern of many groups.

The value of language and traditions is affirmed in many of the chapters in this book, and is especially prominent in treatments by Maje and Maje Raider, and Morgan, and also implicit in the contribution by DeWitt. The health significance of these values also surfaces in a surprising context: the chapter by Oster and his co-authors (Chapter 11) that examines factors affecting diabetes incidence in Cree communities in Alberta. Authors Oster and Toth were based at the University of Alberta medical school and worked with community collaborators, seeking to address one of the most severe health challenges faced by Indigenous communities in much of Canada: diabetes. The extremely high incidence of diabetes, and high rates of serious side effects from the condition in Indigenous communities, is noteworthy, and represents a challenge on numerous levels. Their findings show that language competence in Indigenous language and participation in cultural Ceremonies acts as a proxy for continuance of traditions and healthy identity and can reduce risks of diabetes for communities. It is also likely that traditional treatments, access to healthy traditional foods, and activity on the land are strong contributors to reduced diabetes risk, though these elements were outside the study design.

Another physician contributor, Salvalaggio (Chapter 12) deals with challenges of providing appropriate community-centred and community-responsive care in an impoverished Alberta urban community with high numbers of Indigenous members. She explicitly addresses reconciliation in her efforts to find effective and respectful paradigms of action research and care that honour Indigenous ways of interacting and respect the perspectives and needs of community participants. She offers advice and an approach to physician colleagues about how to implement a community-based research and treatment program, and describes the complementarity of a range of approaches, including harm reduction models that aim for positive interventions concurrently with increasing knowledge of community health issues.

Finally, the introductory contribution by Cree Elder and ceremonialist Harry Watchmaker affirms the deep importance of a spiritually based foundation and of Ceremony. A strong spiritual base aids in seeking and maintaining health in all arenas, and for combatting the multiple effects of trauma and marginalization, especially with regard to the effects of residential schools on survivors and on their communities.

Together these efforts show a range of ways to approach community wellbeing in a collaborative manner. Respect and co-creation of knowledge, which can then inform culturally acceptable practice, is key. However, consistent and adequate funding remains a challenge for many of these initiatives. As Dr. Wilton Littlechild emphasized in his address to the Integrative Health Institute at the University of Alberta in 2017, supporting these efforts and supporting Aboriginal/Indigenous-run programs is an important recommendation of the Canadian Truth and Reconciliation Commission. Successful models of collaborative work to improve and support Indigenous community health must address many structural problems, and must provide adequate funding on a continuing basis to be able to substantially improve the overall picture of Indigenous health in Canada and in Alaska. (The fate of the Aboriginal Healing Foundation in Canada provides a cautionary tale regarding funding stability.) These efforts need more than lip service, and need to be more than the political correctness of the moment, if they are to effectively redress past wrongs and establish a just foundation for collaborative improvement of Indigenous health and well-being.

It is also evident that the maintenance of traditional ways of healing and Traditional Knowledge requires effective transmission of both knowledge and practice (e.g., Robbins and Dewar 2011). Maintaining these is tied up with the health of languages and of the Land, access to intact lands, and valorizing these traditional practices. Effective collaboration in the enterprise of supporting health and community well-being requires going beyond lip service to finding ways forward that blend the wisdom and skills of the past with the potential and new tools available today.

Among the challenging issues that must be faced is how to enable sustainable economic development in rural areas that are Indigenous homelands without compromising the integrity of the land itself and the future of the planet. Poverty remains a significant cause of health issues and challenges to well-being in Indigenous communities. Addressing root causes of the social and economic inequity faced by many Indigenous Peoples is thus key (cf. Kirmayer, Gone, and Moses 2014). The Truth and Reconciliation Commission and the United Nations Declaration on the Rights of Indigenous Peoples lay down the challenge. Now communities, healers, and biomedicine need to work together to craft solutions.

Despite many challenges, the vibrancy and determination of the contributors to forge effective and sustainable and healthy futures for their communities, and the communities with whom they work, stands out, as does the creative blending of many pathways to wholeness and well-being.

NOTE

1.   SRT is an approach to trauma therapy. See the Canadian Foundation for Trauma
      Research information site on SRT at https://www.cftre.com/courses-seminars/
      what-is-self-regulation-therapy/.

REFERENCES

Geddes, G. 2017. *Medicine Unbundled: A Journey through the Minefields of Indigenous Health Care.* Victoria: Heritage House.

Kirmayer, L.J., J.P. Gone, and J. Moses. 2014. "Rethinking Historical Trauma." *Transcultural Psychiatry* 51, no. 3: 299–319.

Moise, M. 2017. *Letter to Cody, the Longest Journey.* Edmonton: Mugo Pine Press Ltd.

Morgan, R.E., compiler. 2016. *Tam Gisst Culture Camp Final Report.* Unpublished report.

Robbins, J.A., and J. Dewar. 2011. "Traditional Indigenous Approaches to Healing and the Modern Welfare of Traditional Knowledge, Spirituality and Lands: A Critical Reflection on Practices and Policies Taken from the Canadian Indigenous Example." *The International Indigenous Policy Journal* 2, no. 4: article 2. http://ir.lib.uwo.ca/iipj/vol2/iss4/2 DOI: 10:18584/iipj.2011.2.4.2.

Contributors

DARLENE P. AUGER is a Nehiyaw and Nahkawiyiniw woman originally from Wabasca, Alberta, who resides in Amiskwâci Wâskahikan (Edmonton). She is a fluent Cree speaker and is passionate about passing on her language through song, story, and healing. Darlene comes from a family of eight, and is a mother of two young ladies, Fawn and Kîstin. Darlene is an educator, researcher, holistic healing practitioner, speaker, actress, singer, and award-winning author of four children's books. Darlene holds a psychology degree from the University of Alberta and a doctoral degree from the University Nuhelotine Thayotsi Nistameyimakanak (Blue Quills, UnBQ) in Iyiniw Pimâtisiwin Kiskeyihtamowin—Indigenous Life Knowledge. She is currently taking the masters of Indigenous social work at UnBQ to develop a program to train therapists in wiwip'son (healing swing) therapy (www.wiwipson.com). She is currently conducting post-doctoral research with the kinesiology and neurology departments at the University of Alberta on the healing swing.

DOROTHY BADRY, PHD, RSW, is a professor in the Faculty of Social Work, University of Calgary. Her research focus is on living with fetal alcohol spectrum disorders (FASD), including child welfare, complex disability and child mental health, women's health and FASD prevention, housing and homelessness, advancing knowledge and training on FASD, loss and grief, and, more recently, FASD and suicide. She is passionate about working in collaboration with rural, remote, and Indigenous communities, and is the child welfare research lead for the Canada Fetal Alcohol Spectrum Disorders Research

Network. Dorothy has been Child Welfare Research Lead since 2017 with the Canada FASD Research Network. She has received numerous research grants from provincial and national funders, including PolicyWise, the Public Health Agency of Canada, the First Nations & Inuit Health Branch of Canada, and Social Sciences and Humanities Research Council. Dorothy served as the co-chair of the Persons with Developmental Disabilities Review in 2019 for the Government of Alberta.

JANELLE MARIE BAKER, PHD, is of European settler and maternal Métis ancestry and is an assistant professor in anthropology at Athabasca University in northern Alberta. She is an ethnobiologist and environmental anthropologist who has collaborated with First Nations on community-based monitoring for industrial contaminants in traditional foods in Treaty No. 8 region since 2006. Janelle is also co-principal investigator with Métis anthropologist Zoe Todd on a project that is restor(y)ing land use governance and bull trout population health in a contested area of the Rocky Mountain foothills in Alberta, which is where Janelle resides with her family. Janelle is the North Americas Representative on the board of directors for the International Society of Ethnobiology and a co-editor of *Ethnobiology Letters*, a gold open-access, online, peer-reviewed journal. She is the winner of the 2019 Canadian Association for Graduate Studies—ProQuest Distinguished Dissertation Award, Arts, Humanities, and Social Sciences category.

MARGARET OLIN HOFFMAN DAVID was born and raised in rural Alaska. She grew up spending summers at her grandparents' fish camp on the Yukon River, and is rooted by her Koyukon Athabascan culture. Through fifteen years of working in tribal and rural community health promotion and program management, birthing her family, volunteering as a doula, and healing through Native ways of knowing, she realized her call to midwifery. The potential to heal ourselves, and our ancestors, during the transformation of childbirth is why she has chosen to dedicate her life's work to midwifery. Through her work as a certified nurse midwife, she hopes to expand perinatal community health programs and birthing options for rural Alaska Native women by remembering traditional practices and supporting more pathways for Indigenous birth workers. She is a founding member of the National Indigenous Midwifery Alliance and the Alaska Native Birthworkers Community. She lives on Dena'ina land in Anchorage, Alaska, with her partner and four children, and is a midwife at the Alaska Native Medical Center.

MEDA DEWITT's Tlingit names are Tśa Tsée Náakw, Khaat kła.at, her adopted Iñupiaq name is Tigigalook, and her adopted Cree name is Boss Eagle Spirit Woman, or "Boss." Her Clan is Naanyaa.aayí, and she is a child of the Kaach.aadi. Her family comes from Shtuxéen kwaan (now referred to as Wrangell, Alaska). Meda's lineage also comes from Oregon, Washington, British Columbia, and Yukon Territory. Currently, she lives on Dena'ina lands in Anchorage, Alaska, with her fiancé James "Chris" Paoli and their eight children. Meda's work revolves around the personal credo, "Leave a world that can support life and a culture worth living for." Her work experience draws from her training as an Alaska Native Traditional Healer and Healthy Native Communities capacity building facilitator.

HAL EAGLETAIL, Tsuut'ina Nation, is a traditional practitioner and follower of Dene spiritual and cultural ways and lifestyle. He is a practitioner of herbal medicines, Pipe Carrier, Sweat Lodge Keeper, and residential school survivor. Hal works for Alberta Health Services to help hospital patients get back to health with Traditional Knowledge of herbs and Ceremony. He is also a master of ceremonies for First Nation powwows and Round Dance celebrations across North America. Hal facilitates conferences and workshops, and has travelled internationally with First Nations dance troupes to help educate and promote First Nations history and cultural identity. He has travelled to New Zealand, Switzerland, Germany, France, and England. In 2007, he was asked by the Alberta government to represent First Nations of Alberta at the Smithsonian Folklife Festival in Washington, DC.

GARY FERGUSON serves as faculty and director of outreach and engagement at Washington State University's Institute for Research and Education to Advance Community Health, located in the Elson S. Floyd College of Medicine. Formally trained as a naturopathic physician, he has a passion for promoting healthy communities with a population health approach. He is Aleut/Unangax, originally from the Shumagin Islands community of Sand Point, Alaska. Gary's past positions include providing clinical services to his home region at Eastern Aleutian Tribes, serving at the Alaska Native Tribal Health Consortium as wellness and prevention director and senior director of community health services, and as chief executive officer at the Rural Alaska Community Action Program. His volunteer work includes serving as chair/board director for the American Indian Cancer Foundation; board director for the Aleut Corporation; commissioner on the National Certification Commission for Addiction Professionals; board director for the Alaska Addiction Professionals Association; member of the Sustainable Development Working Group, Arctic Human Health Expert Group, on behalf of the Aleut International Association; and committee member on University of Alaska's Master of Pubic Health Advisory Committee. See www.drgaryferguson.com.

MARC FONDA held an adjunct research professorship in sociology at Western University at the time of writing his chapter. He is presently a private scholar. He has had a long career supporting and conducting policy-relevant research, both at the Social Sciences and Humanities Research Council of Canada and at what is now Indigenous Services Canada. Among his contributions are helping establish and manage the *International Indigenous Policy Journal*, acting as the managing editor of the second volume of *Hidden in Plain Sight* (Newhouse, Voyager and Beavon, 2011), and has published several articles on the well-being impacts of revitalizing Indigenous traditional cultures.

ANNIE I. (NIPALAYOK) GOOSE was born in the summer of July 1948 in Minto Inlet to Sam and Rene Oliktoak. She was adopted by Jacob Nipalayuk, an Alaskan Inupiat, and his wife, Agnes Nigiyok. Annie is fluent in Inuinaqtun and Inuvialuktun. In the 1950s, Annie attended residential schools in Coppermine

(Kugluktuk, Nunavut) and Inuvik, Northwest Territories. She married William (Billy) Kayutak Goose on September 6, 1966, in Holman (Ulukhaktok, Northwest Territories). They had six children and adopted a boy from Inuvik, Northwest Territories. Annie has worked in social work, government field service, Aboriginal land claims and self-government, healing and wellness, cultural and traditional program delivery, and alcohol and drug counselling. Annie has contributed to many organizations, boards, and projects, and in 2012 she was the recipient of the Woman of the Year award for Pauktuutiit Inuit Women of Canada. Her hobbies are sewing, taking walks along the beach, and spending time outdoors with her family, children, and grandchildren whenever possible. In her own journey of self-healing, she has led a sober life for twenty-seven years and hopes to see healthier and more self-reliant Aboriginal people of the North. Annie has twenty or so grandchildren, and lives in Ulukhaktok, Northwest Territories.

ANGELA GRIER, PIIOHKSOOPANSKII/ SINGING LOUDLY FAR AWAY (Piikani/ Blackfoot), M.Ed., is a registered provisional psychologist and the Indigenous initiatives lead for the Canadian Counselling and Psychotherapy Association. Her graduate research explored Blackfoot and Indigenous psychology and methodologies. She has over twenty-five years of experience as a First Nation/Indigenous direct and systemic advocate, which includes areas of Indigenous psychology, child rights, post-secondary education, leadership, community development, and Blackfoot ways of knowing. She is a proud mother and grandmother to Meadow.

LESLIE MAIN JOHNSON, PHD, is professor emerita at Athabasca University. She is an ethnographer and ethnobiologist who works with Indigenous Peoples in northwestern Canada. Her work has explored ethnobiology, knowledge of the land, and traditional medicines and healing. She is also fascinated by people's stories, and by skills required to make traditional artifacts. She is editor of *Wisdom Engaged: Traditional Knowledge for Northern Community Well-Being* (Polynya Press, 2019), author of *Trail of Story, Traveller's Path: Reflections on Ethnoecology and Landscape*

(Athabasca University Press, 2010), and co-editor of *Landscape Ethnoecology: Concepts of Biotic and Physical Space*, with Eugene S. Hunn (Berghan Books, 2010). Her dissertation, *Health, Wholeness and the Land: Gitksan Traditional Plant Use and Healing*, is in demand in Gitxsan communities, where some six hundred hardbound copies have been distributed. Her present research is on the history and design of Indigenous snowshoes in northwestern North America. She is also a mother and grandmother, and enjoys spending time with her family.

ALLISON KELLIHER, MD, is the first Koyukon Athabascan physician, King Salmon Clan, from Nome, Alaska. She was trained as a Traditional Healer since childhood, and has studied and apprenticed with other healers globally. She is the only physician trained as a Tribal Doctor in Alaska's health system. She directs the American Indian Collaborative Research Network at the University of North Dakota School of Medicine and Health Sciences. She is also an assistant professor in the Department of Family & Community Medicine. She serves as director-at-large for the Association of American Indian Physicians. She is board certified in family medicine and integrative and holistic medicine.

RICK LIGHTNING is an Elder/Mosom from Maskwacis, raised in the traditions of Nehiyaw (Plains Cree). He is a third-generation residential school survivor. Through his consulting company, Lightning Camp and Associates, Rick has facilitated cross-cultural training, youth workshops, grief recovery, and program assessments. He is certified as a mental health therapist/counsellor trained in suicide and gang intervention. Rick also has mediation, negotiation, and restorative justice certification. As a policy technician, he has assisted with the United Nations Declaration on the Rights of Indigenous Peoples. He has also been a cultural advisor to Truth and Reconciliation Commissioner Wilton J. Littlechild. Rick has been a cultural support worker to the Indian Residential Schools, Mental Health, and Aboriginal Youth Communities Empowerment Strategy, and the National Native Alcohol and Drug Abuse Program at Maskwacis. Currently, Rick is the resident Elder, or Mosom, as he prefers to be called, for the Faculty of Medicine and Dentistry, University of Alberta.

MARY MAJE is a Kaska Elder from Ross River, Yukon. She is fluent in her language. She has been involved with the Liard Aboriginal Women's Society since its founding, and has served on its board. She is also active in efforts to care for the land, and has been involved with resource development response in the Ross River area. She continues to spend time on the Land, especially in her cabin along the Robert Campbell Highway south of Ross River.

ANN MAJE RAIDER is a Kaska grandmother and social justice advocate. Following her service as the first democratically elected Chief of the Liard First Nation from 1992 to 1998, Ann engaged with a small group of Kaska women to create the Liard Aboriginal Women's Society (LAWS). Committed to addressing the legacy of colonialism, the society created a multi-year healing strategy aimed at responding to the physical and sexual abuse that occurred at residential schools. In recent years, LAWS and the RCMP have implemented a community safety protocol (Together for Justice), and recently unveiled two new multi-year initiatives—a Youth for Safety Project and Women's Advocacy Service. Ann has served on the Yukon Advisory Council on Women's Issues (2006–2016) and the Yukon Aboriginal Women's Circle (2000–2004). She is a recipient of the 2017 Governor General Polar Award for her leadership. She is also the recipient of the Yukon Government Community Safety Award for Outstanding Project in 2016 for her work on Together for Justice.

MARIA J. MAYAN is a professor in the School of Public Health at the University of Alberta and an associate director of the Community-University Partnership. She is an engaged scholar who situates her work at the intersection of government, not-for-profit, disadvantaged, and clinician communities. She grounds her work in the policy environment, and focuses on how we can work together on complex health and social issues. Her work focuses on the causes of marginalization and how to mobilize against systems of inequity, using primarily qualitative and community-engaged research in rigorous and creative ways. Her qualitative expertise has culminated into a book, *Essentials of Qualitative Inquiry* (Routledge, 2009).

RUBY E. MORGAN, LUU GISS YEE, is a Gitxsan woman of the Gitwangak̲ G̲aneda, Gitxsan Nation. She is passionate about upholding traditional ethics and values in a modern context, and has dedicated herself to supporting and bettering the health and well-being of her community. The community is guided by Matriarchs, and has traditional governance and values, creating a strong community infrastructure. By realizing their inheritance as a community, Gixsan can create a better world, in the spirit of truth and reconciliation, to return the Laxyip (territories) to a place of healing. *T'yoo yaxsi'y 'niin.*

RICHARD T. OSTER, PHD, lives in Edmonton, Alberta, Treaty Six Territory and Métis Region Four, Canada. His ceremonial name, given to him by Mosom Rick Lightning, of Ermineskin Cree Nation, Maskwacis, is Wâpastim (White Horse). Richard comes from mixed European descent, including Danish, Scottish, German, Austrian, and Ukrainian. His family has lived in this area for four generations. He is the scientific director for the Indigenous Wellness Core of Alberta Health Services. He is also an adjunct assistant professor in both the Department of Agricultural, Food and Nutritional Science (University of Alberta) and the Department of Community Health Sciences (University of Calgary). Richard is immersed in Indigenous health, and his academic research program takes a strengths-based and relationship-based approach, building specifically on Indigenous ways of knowing and the resilience and strength within communities.

CAMILLE (PABLO) RUSSELL, SHOOTING IN THE AIR, was born on the Blood Reserve in southern Alberta. He grew up very close to his grandparents, where he learned about his roots and traditions. Following his own Vision Quests, he spent eighteen years in Europe before returning home to help his people as a support worker for the Indian Residential Schools (IRS), an IRS Elder with Treaty 7 Management Corp., a spiritual counsellor at the Elbow River Healing Lodge, and as a Native coordinator at the Calgary Remand Centre. "All healing, all thanks goes to the Creator. He doctors," says Pablo. Over the past twenty years, he has lectured based on the principle of "Follow the Buffalo." The buffalo represents to Native people the qualities of perseverance, facing the storms of life, and walking into them. Pablo received commendation from the government for teaching Blackfoot culture to thirty-two thousand students at the Glenbow Museum in one year. He is also a recipient of the City of Calgary's Chief David Crowchild Memorial Award. Pablo has written *The Path of the Buffalo Medicine Wheel* (ETNA Edition, 2014).

GINETTA SALVALAGGIO, MD MSC CCFP (AM), is an associate professor in the University of Alberta Department of Family Medicine, and the associate scientific director of the Inner City Health and Wellness Program. She received her degree in medicine from the University of Alberta, and completed a family practice residency in Thunder Bay, Ontario. Initially practising as a rural locum, she eventually returned to Edmonton to establish a maternity care and family practice. Dr. Salvalaggio joined the Department of Family Medicine in 2007. She has also completed a masters of science in population health through the University of Alberta School of Public Health. Her academic interests are focused on social accountability, patient and community engagement, and health services for urban underserved populations.

ELLEN L. TOTH joined the faculty at the University of Alberta and University of Alberta Hospital in 1986. Throughout her clinical and research career, Ellen's efforts were in the field of diabetes. Since retirement from the Department of Medicine, she has concentrated on medical care for Indigenous Peoples and communities. She previously studied the incidence and prevalence of diabetes in First Nations, and directed the implementation of the SLICK project, which addressed the complications of diabetes in First Nations communities in Alberta from 2001 to 2011. She also directed MDSI: Mobile Diabetes Screening Initiative, a project funded by Alberta Health and Wellness that went to Aboriginal off-reserve and remote communities, screening for diabetes, until 2014. Since 2009, Ellen has worked for Alberta Health Services in a leadership position in Indigenous health. She is the medical lead for an Aboriginal Wellness ARP (alternate relationship program), involving approximately fifty practitioners in Aboriginal communities.

HAROLD (HARRY) WATCHMAKER is a Cree Nation Knowledge Keeper from Kehewin Cree Nation. He believes deeply in living a spiritual life through Ceremony and raising his family. He has served as a cultural support to the Indian Residential School Resolution Health Support team for the duration of the Truth and Reconciliation Commission, and continues to culturally support individuals, communities, agencies, and industries across Canada. Harry has worked as an advisory Elder with groups such as Tribal Chief Ventures Inc., Bent Arrow Traditional Healing Society, Boyle Street Community Services, and many others. In addition to his community work, Harry is knowledgeable and experienced in the areas of the Sundance, Horse Dance, Chicken Dance, and the Sweat Lodge Ceremony (among other Ceremonies). Harry believes it is his duty to share, support, and remind Canadians about the traditional teachings and practices he has received from his Elders and other communities.

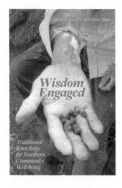

Wisdom Engaged

Traditional Knowledge for Northern Community Well-Being

Patterns of Northern Traditional Healing Series, volume 3

LESLIE MAIN JOHNSON

Collaboration between traditional knowledge and Western bio-medicine aims to improve health care in Northern communities.

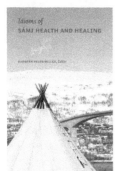

Idioms of Sámi Health and Healing

Patterns of Northern Traditional Healing Series, volume 2

BARBARA HELEN MILLER

Ten experts document the strength of local communities' using traditional resources for health and prevention.

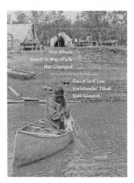

Our Whole Gwich'in Way of Life Has Changed / Gwich'in K'yuu Gwiidandài' Tthak Ejuk Gòonlih

Stories from the People of the Land

LESLIE MCCARTNEY & GWICH'IN TRIBAL COUNCIL

Life-stories of 23 Gwich'in Elders from the Northwest Territories in Canada speak to changing times.

More information at uap.ualberta.ca

CPSIA information can be obtained
at www.ICGtesting.com
Printed in the USA
JSHW020730170523
41827JS00003B/16